I0787687

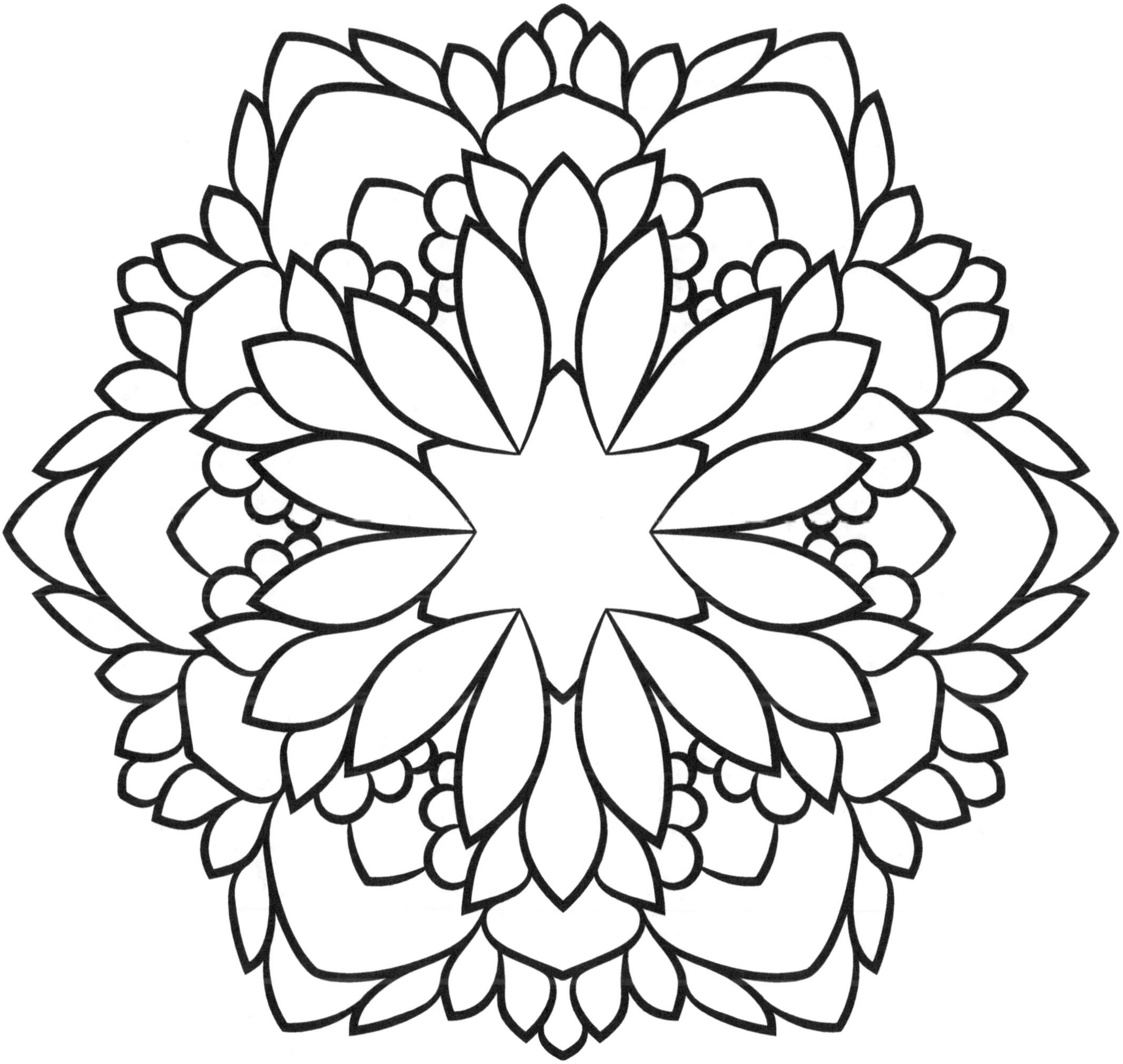

COLORING BOOK

by Little Mary

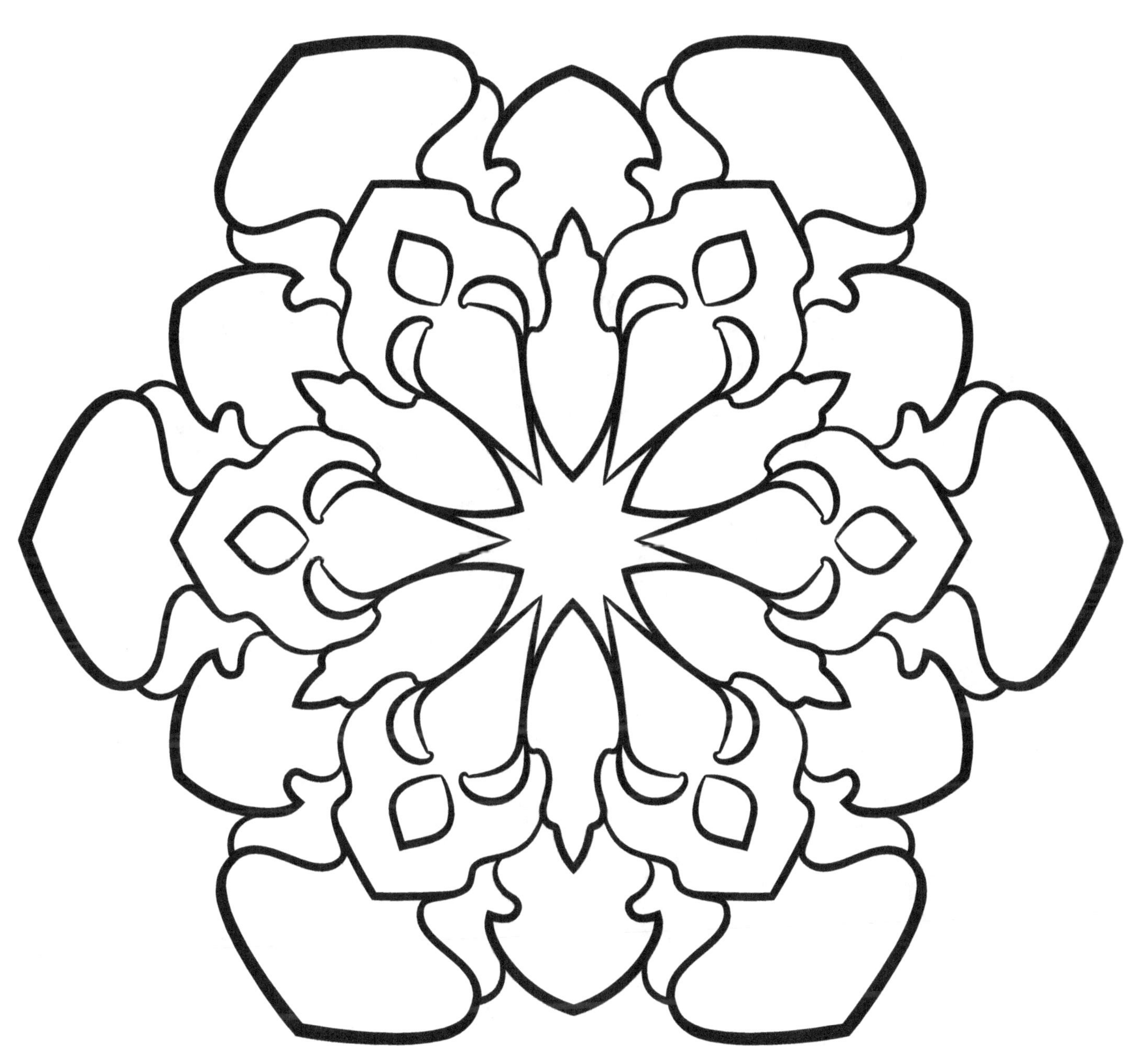

COLORING BOOK

by Little Mary

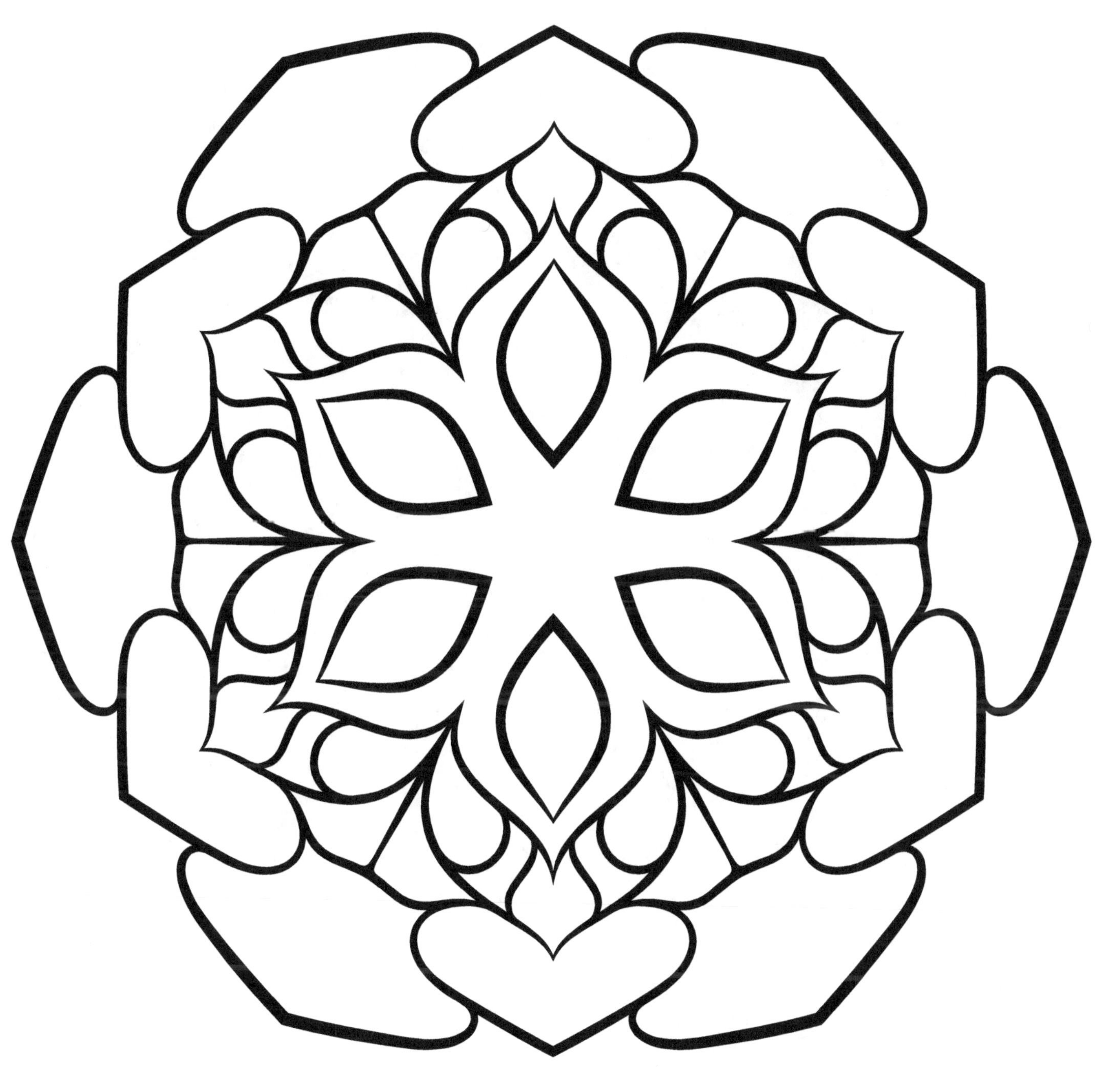

COLORING BOOK

by Little Mary

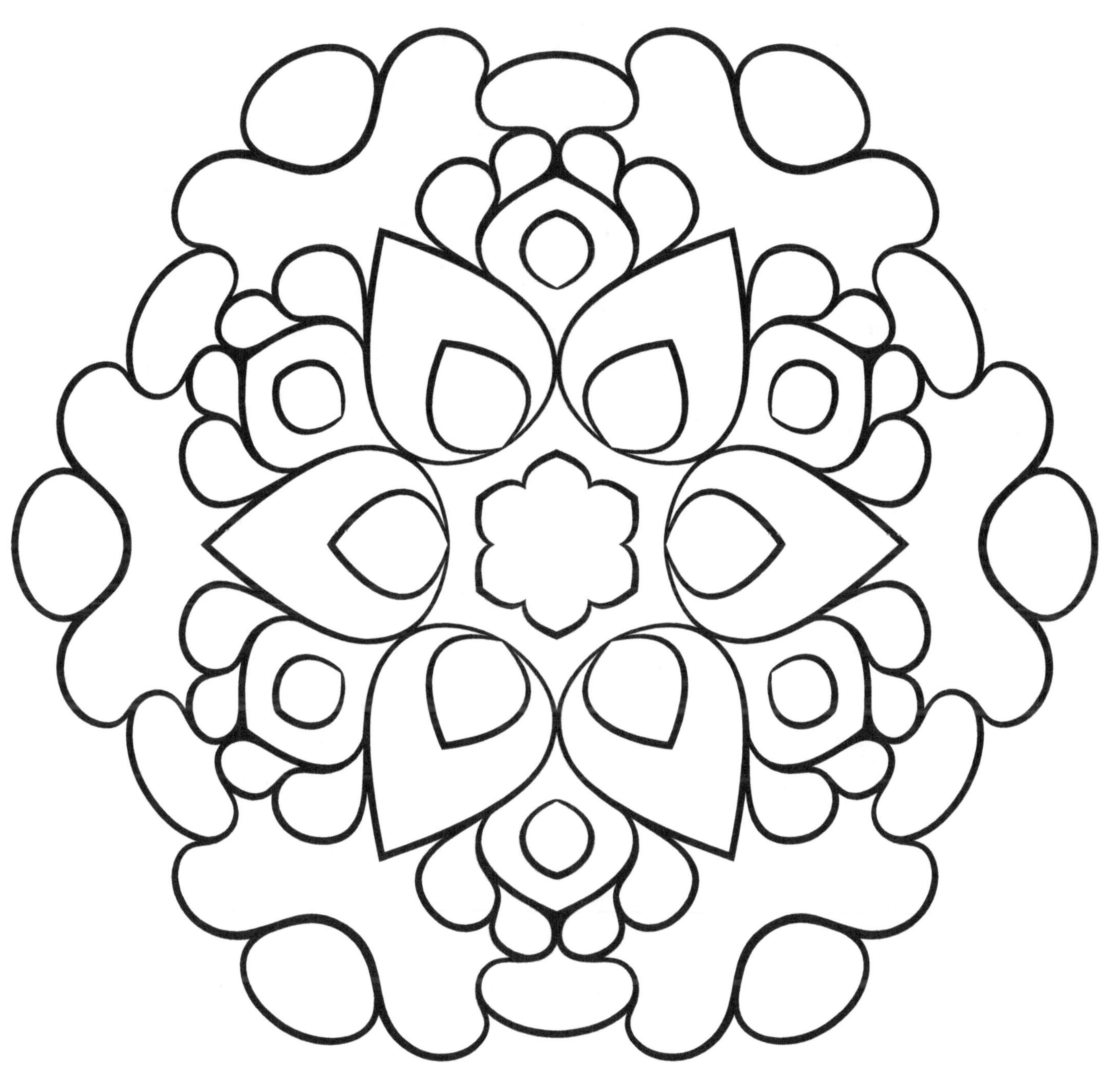

COLORING BOOK

by Little Mary

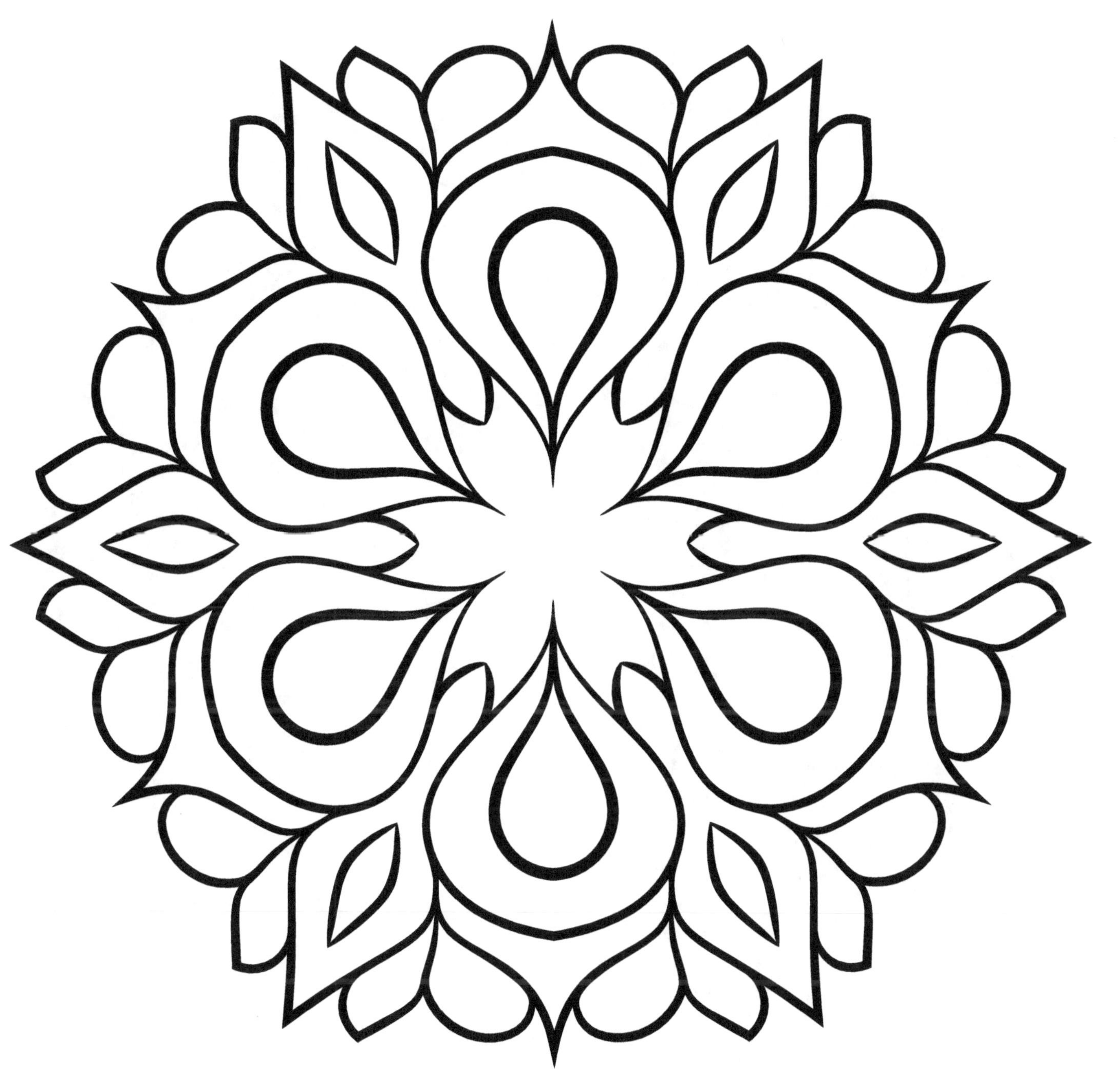

COLORING BOOK

by Little Mary

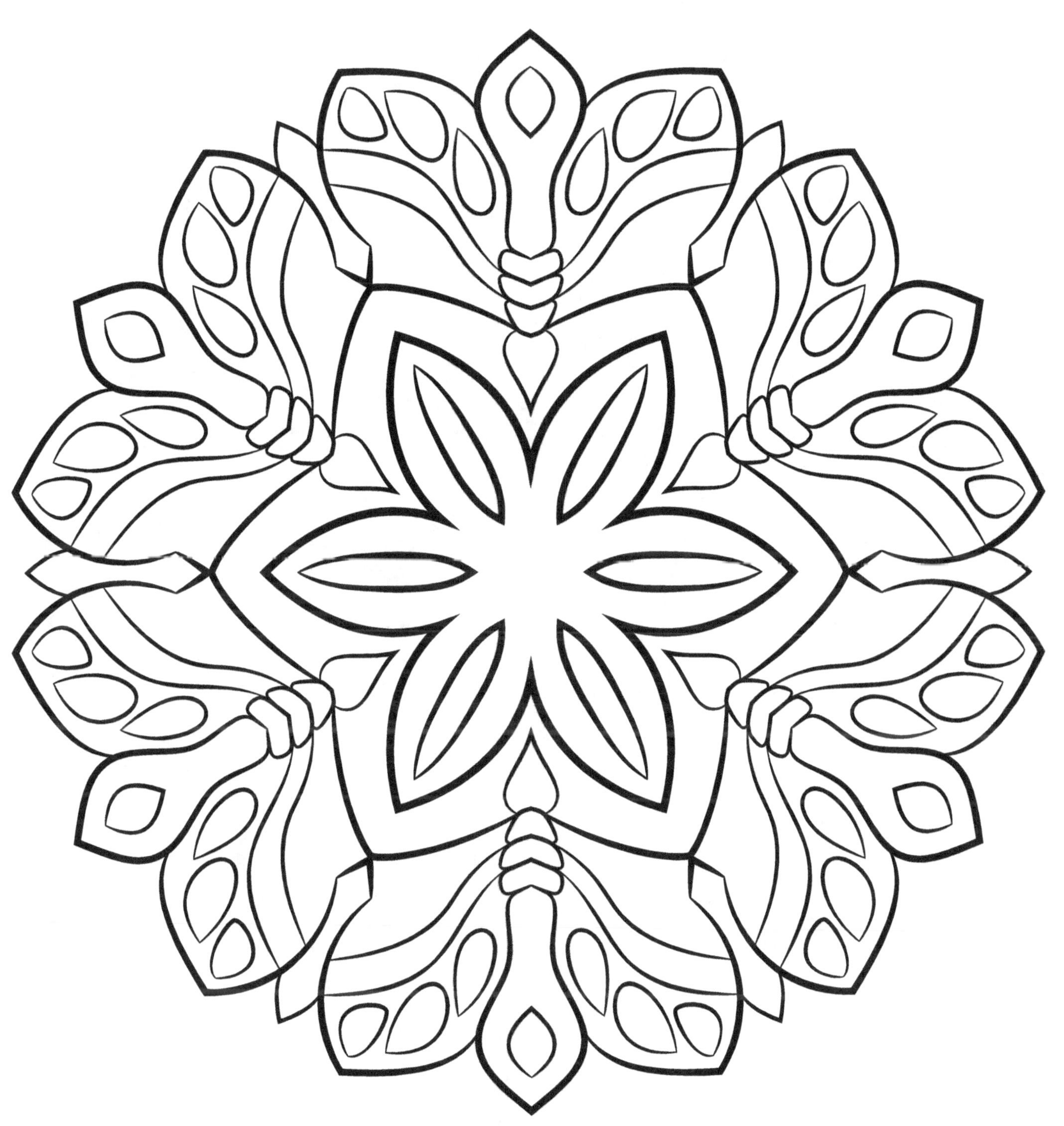

COLORING BOOK

by Little Mary

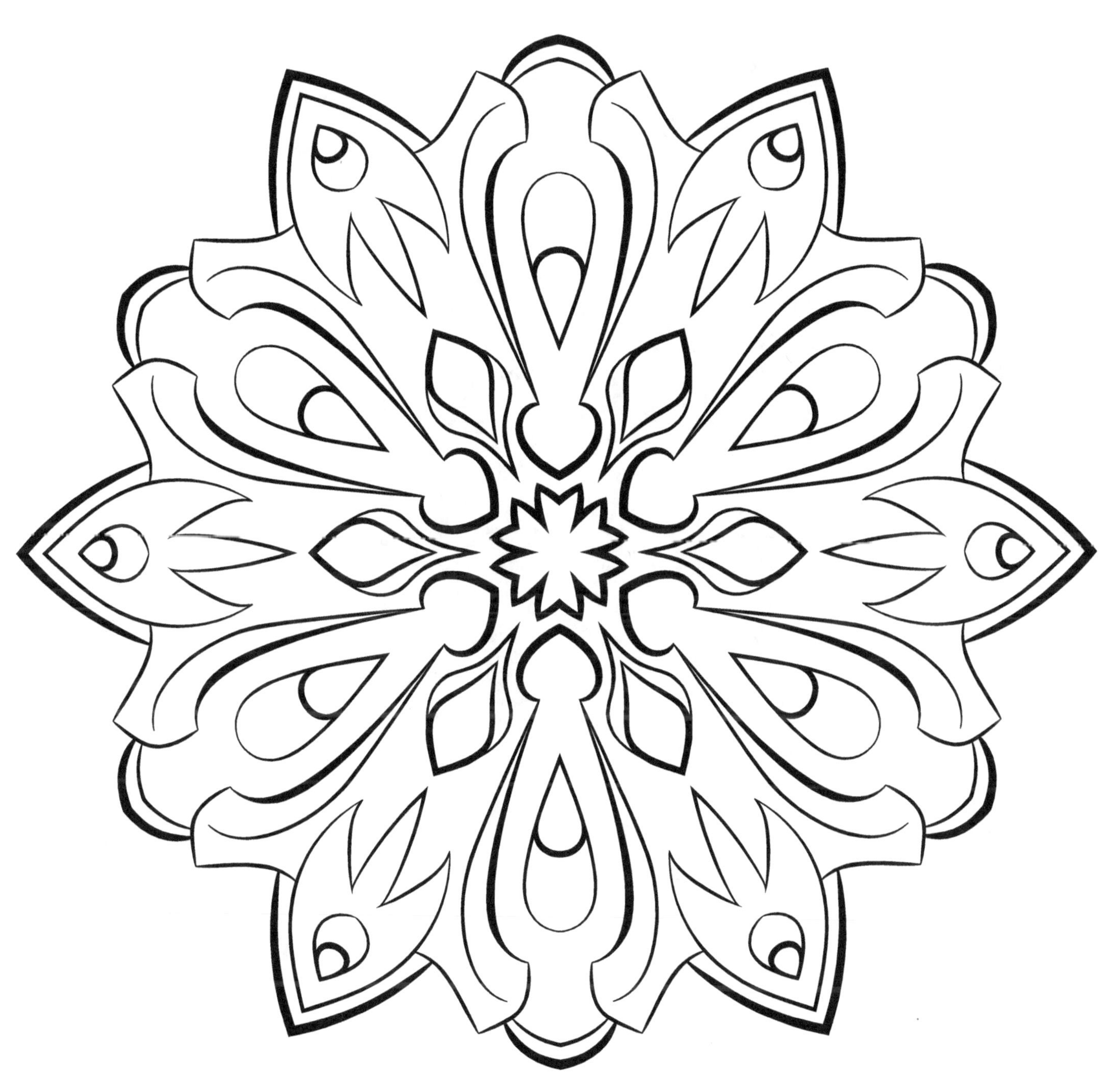

COLORING BOOK

by Little Mary

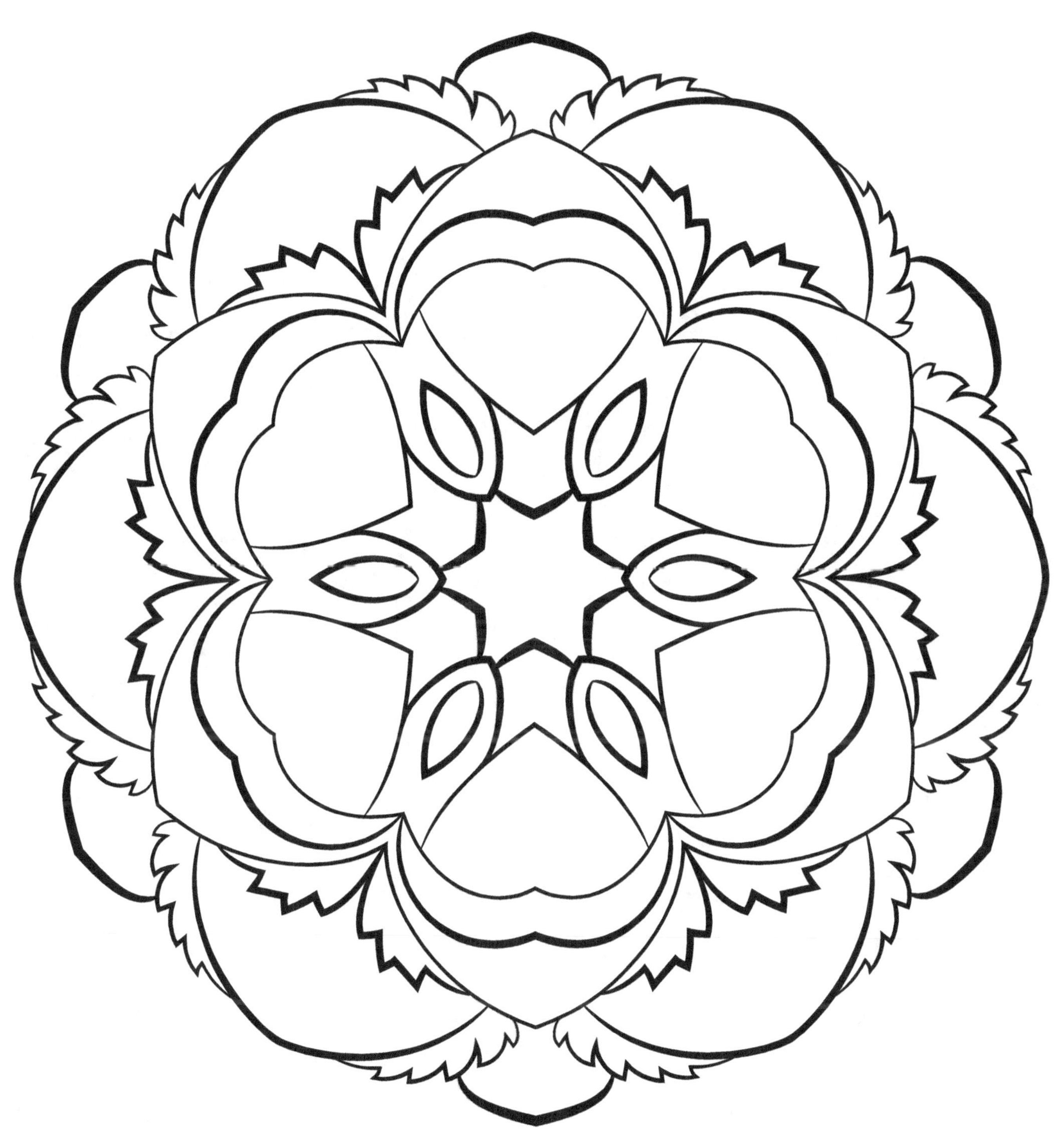

COLORING BOOK

by Little Mary

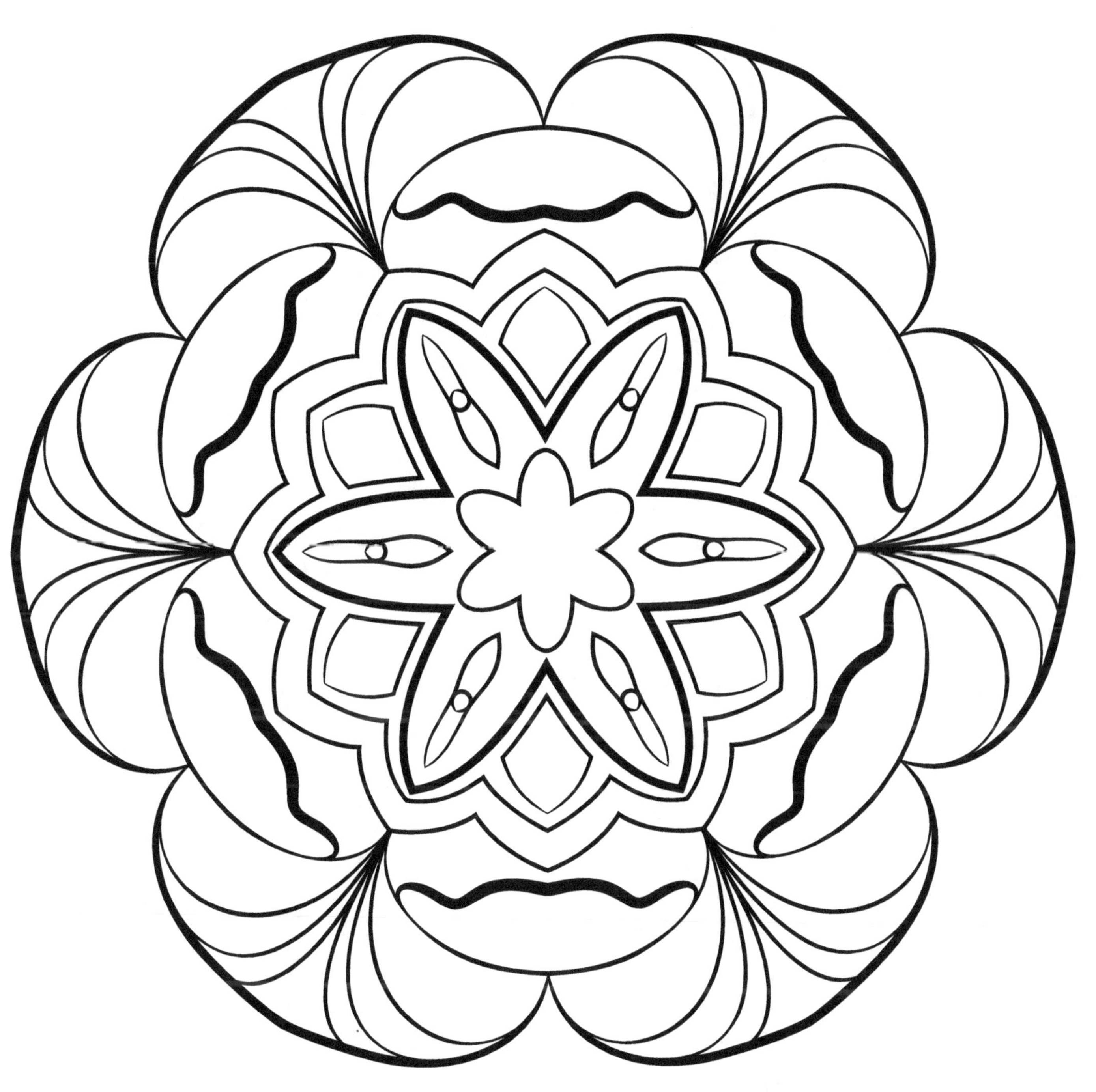

COLORING BOOK

by Little Mary

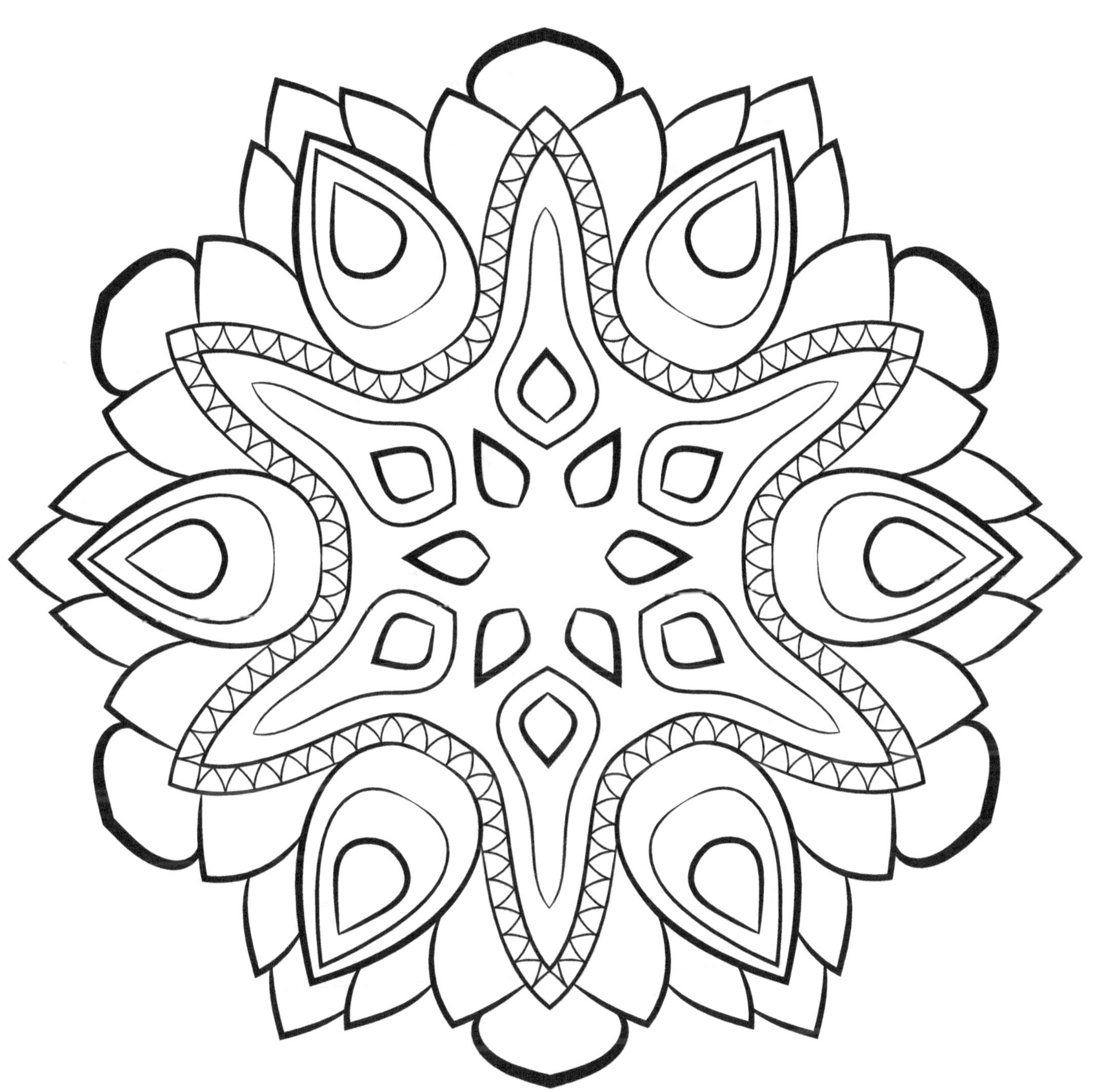

COLORING BOOK

by Little Mary

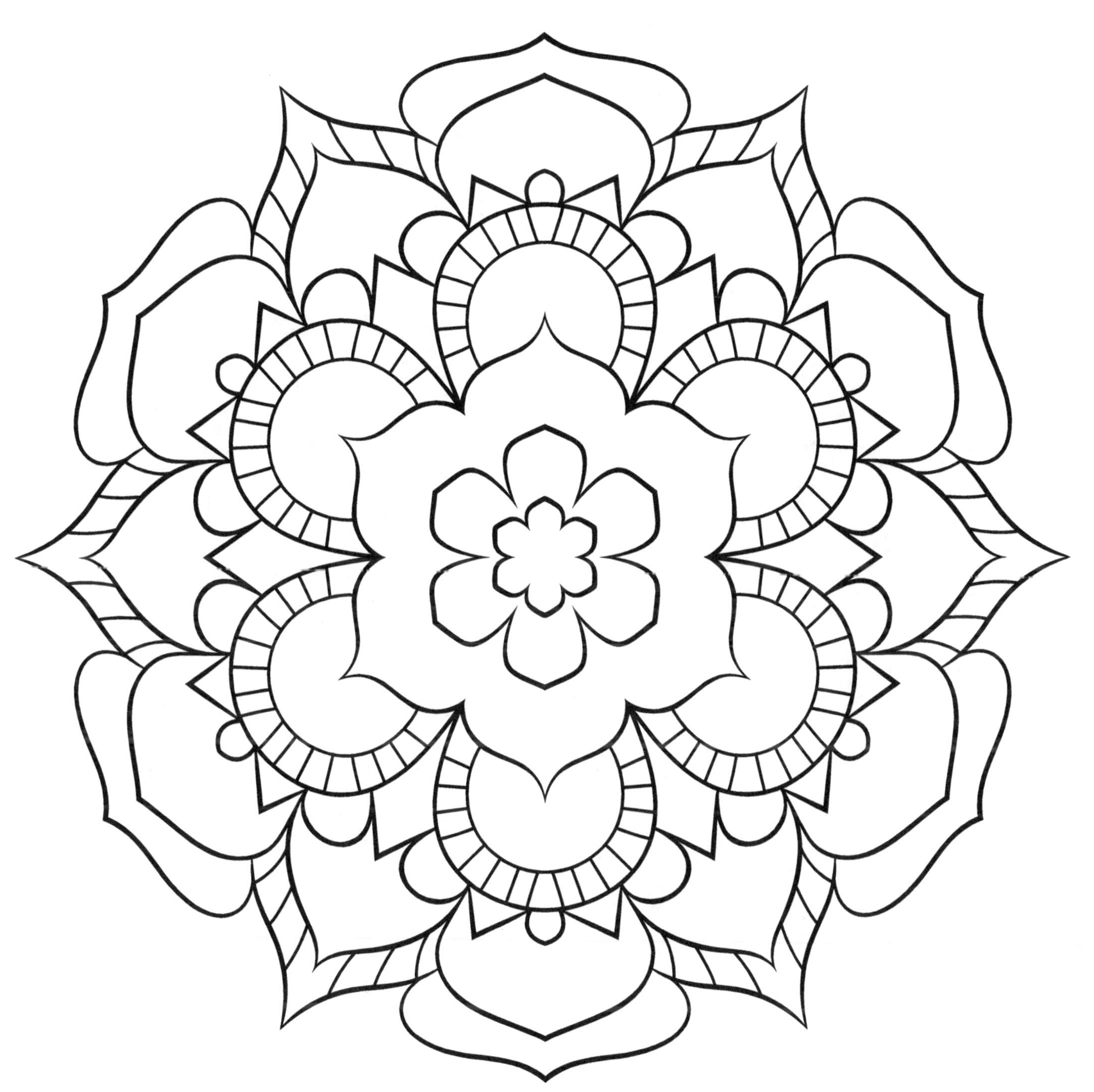

COLORING BOOK

by Little Mary

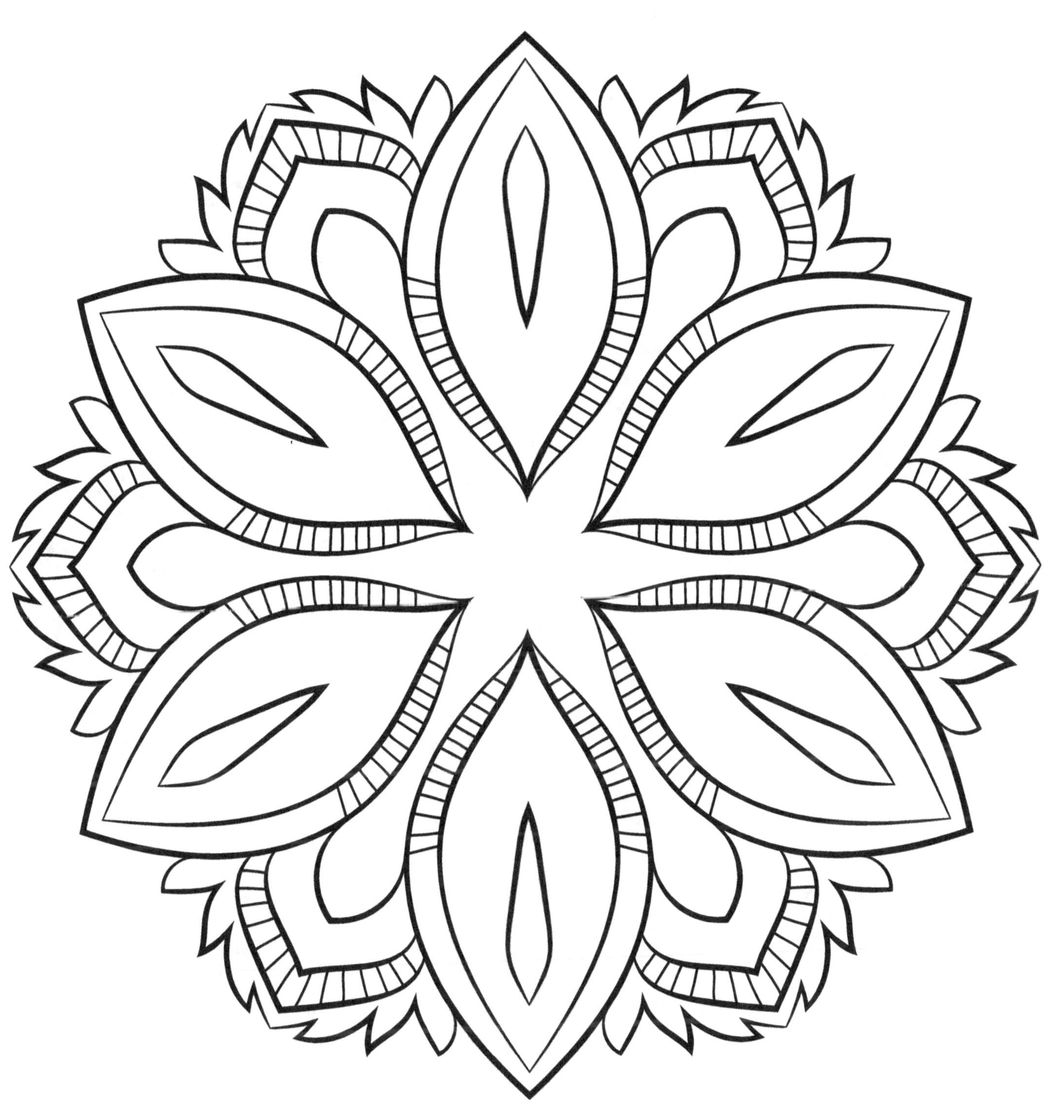

COLORING BOOK

by Little Mary

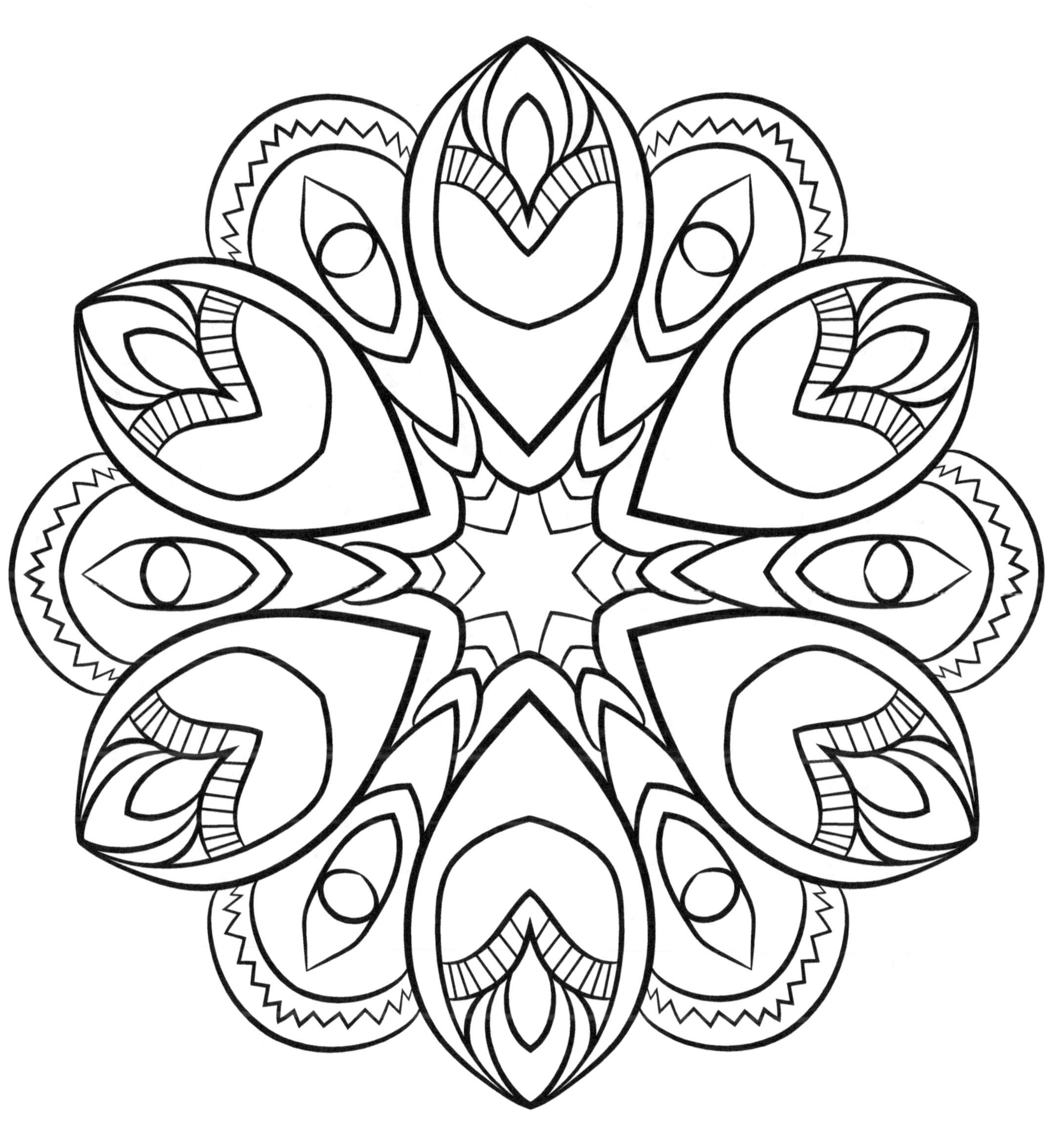

COLORING BOOK

by Little Mary

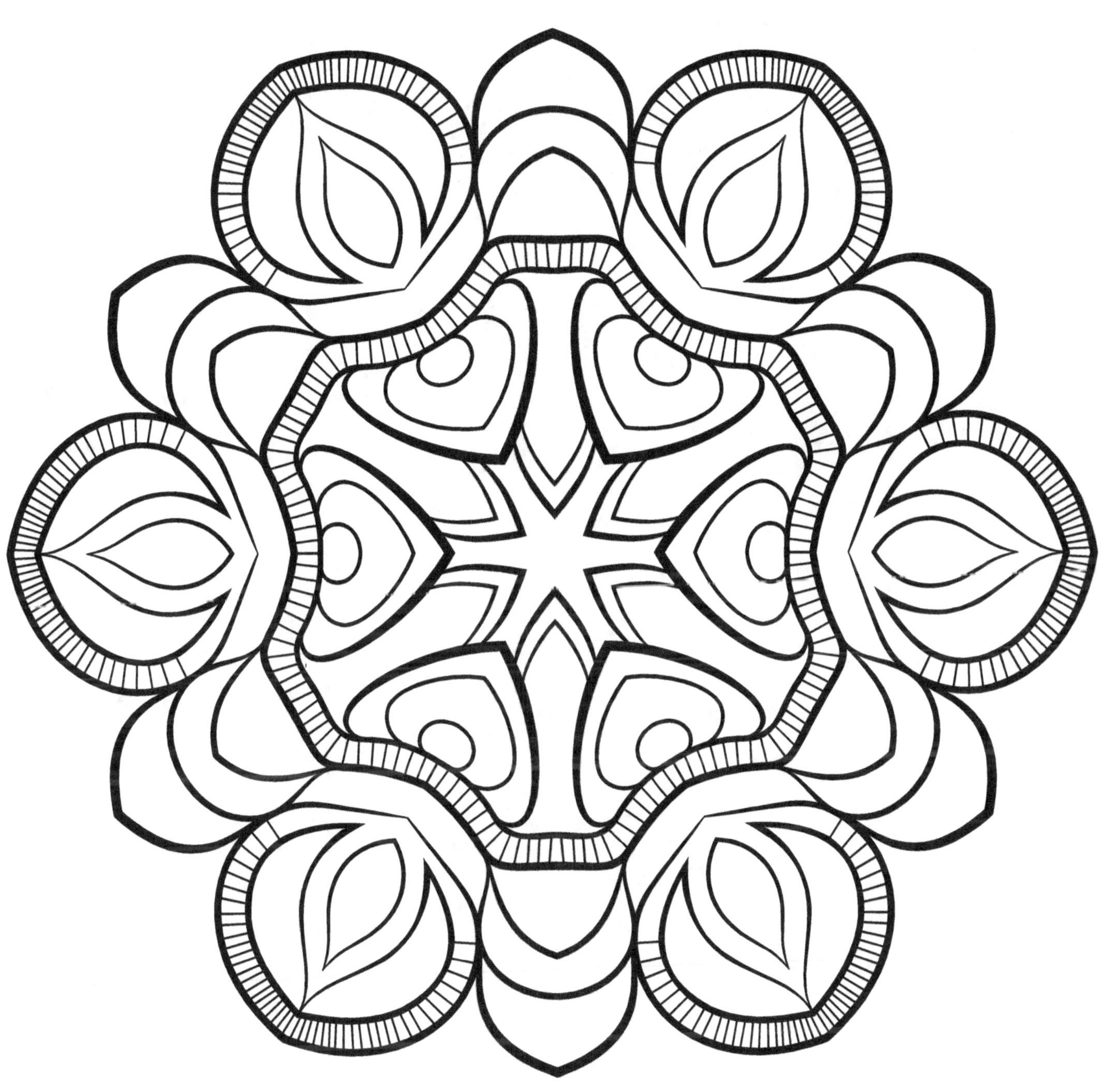

COLORING BOOK

by Little Mary

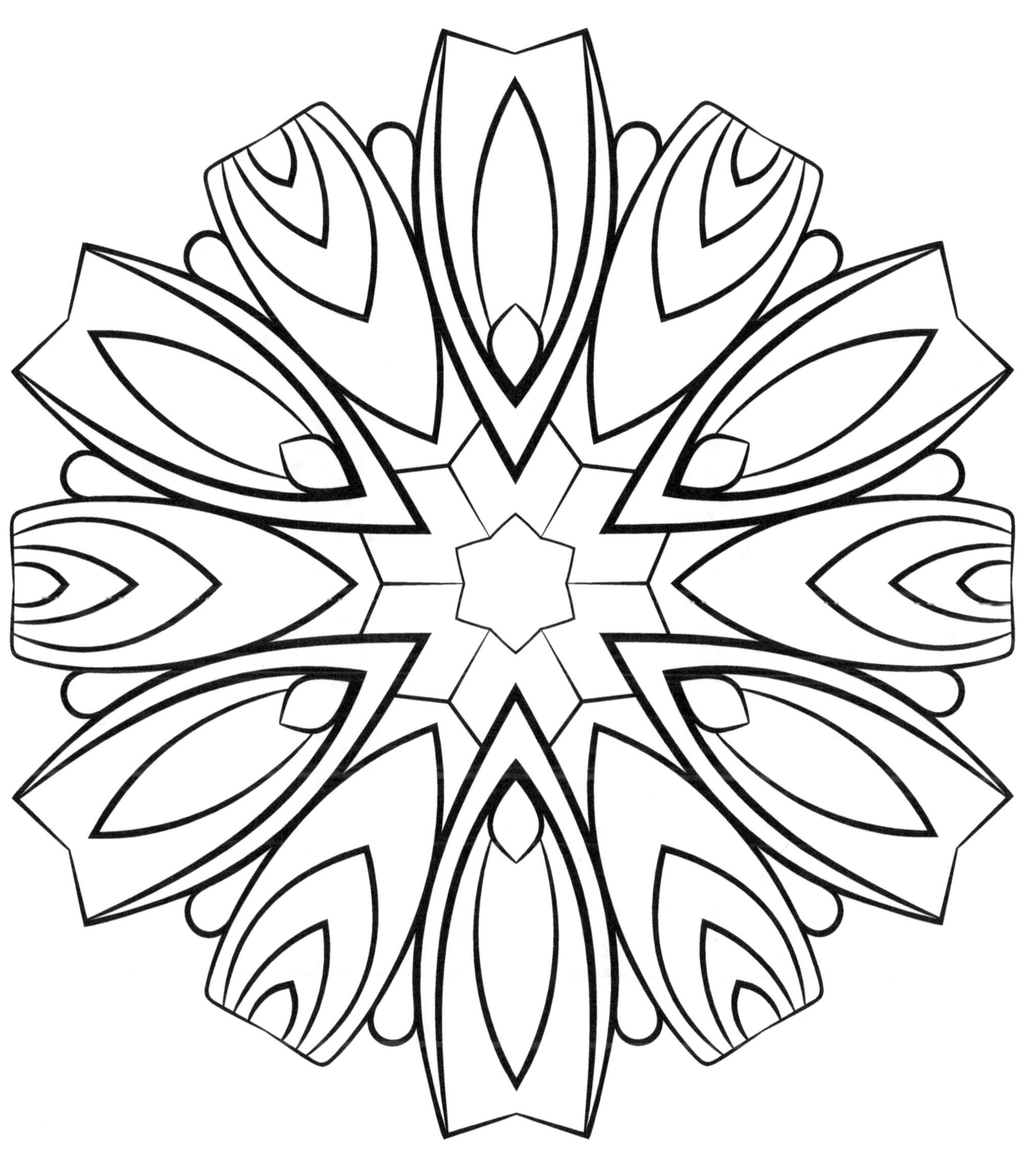

COLORING BOOK

by Little Mary

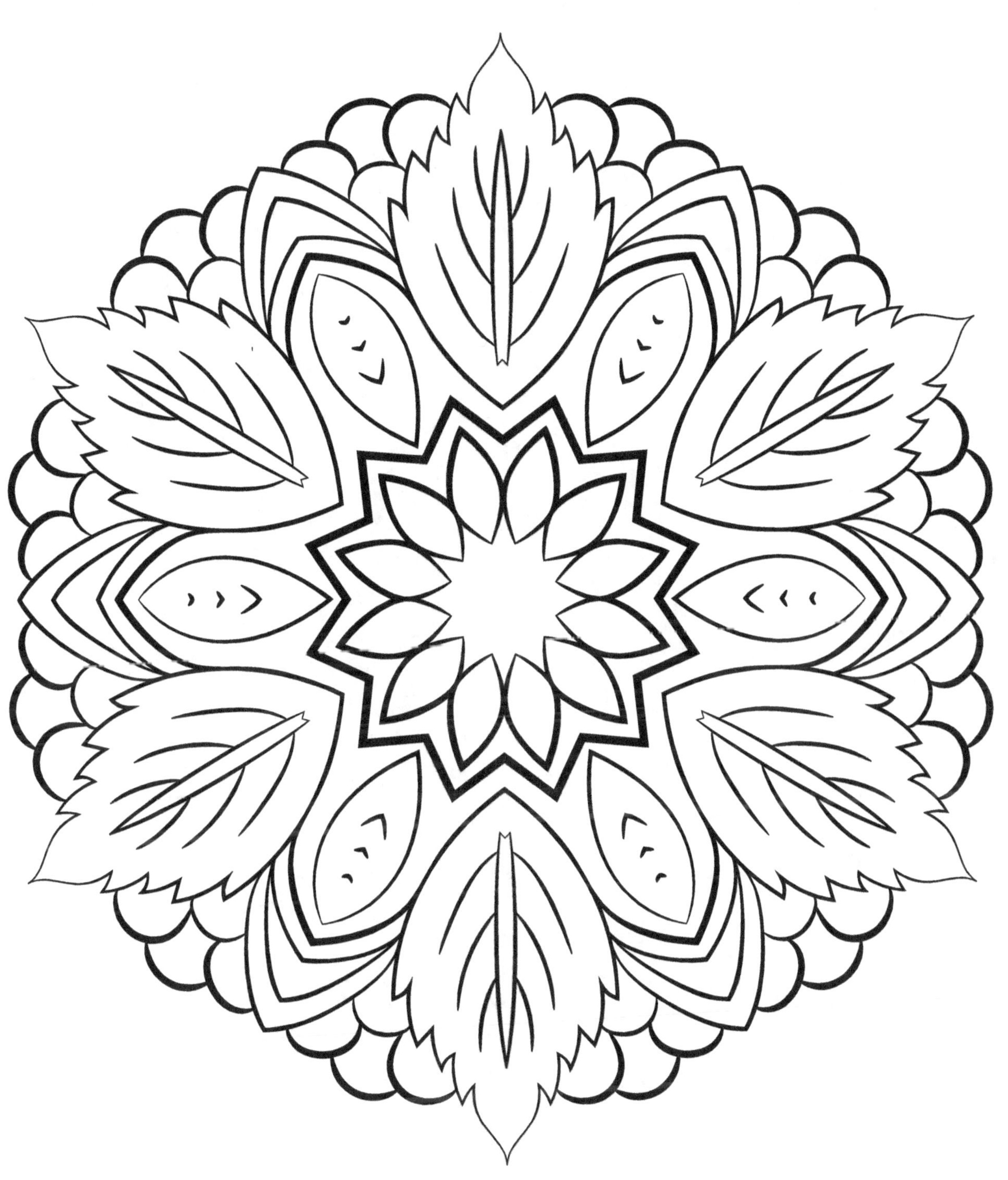

COLORING BOOK

by Little Mary

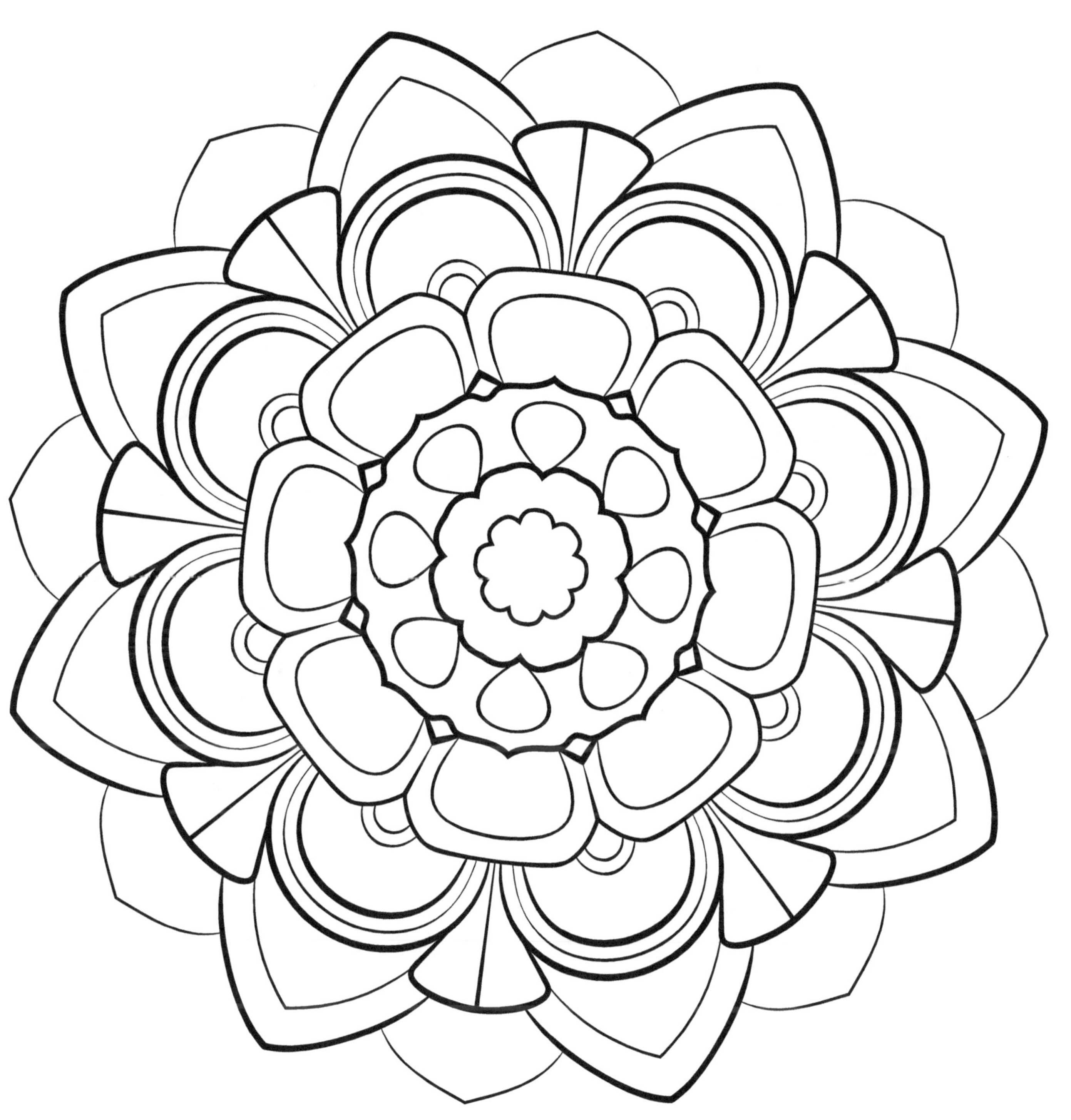

COLORING BOOK

by Little Mary

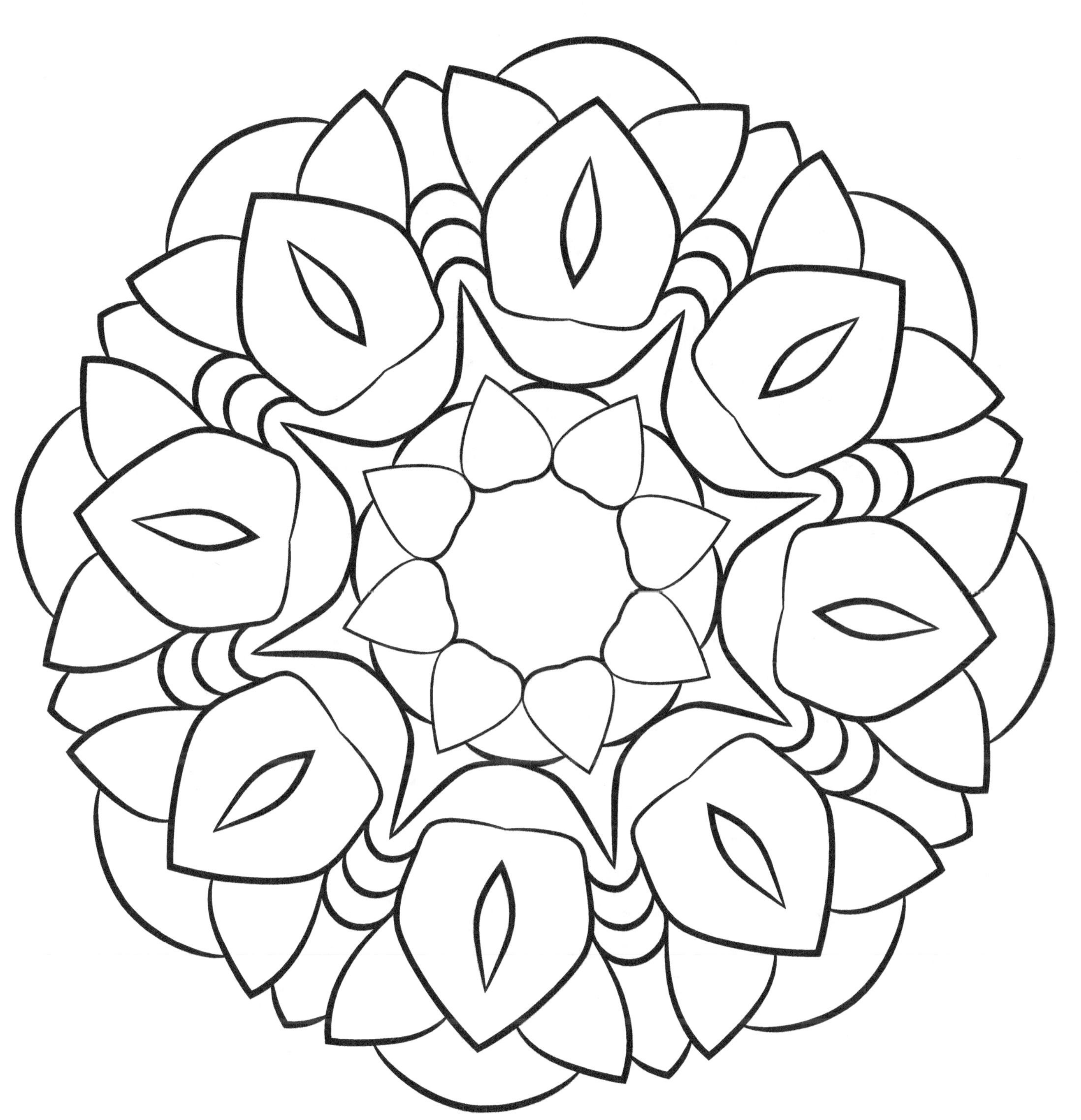

COLORING BOOK

by Little Mary

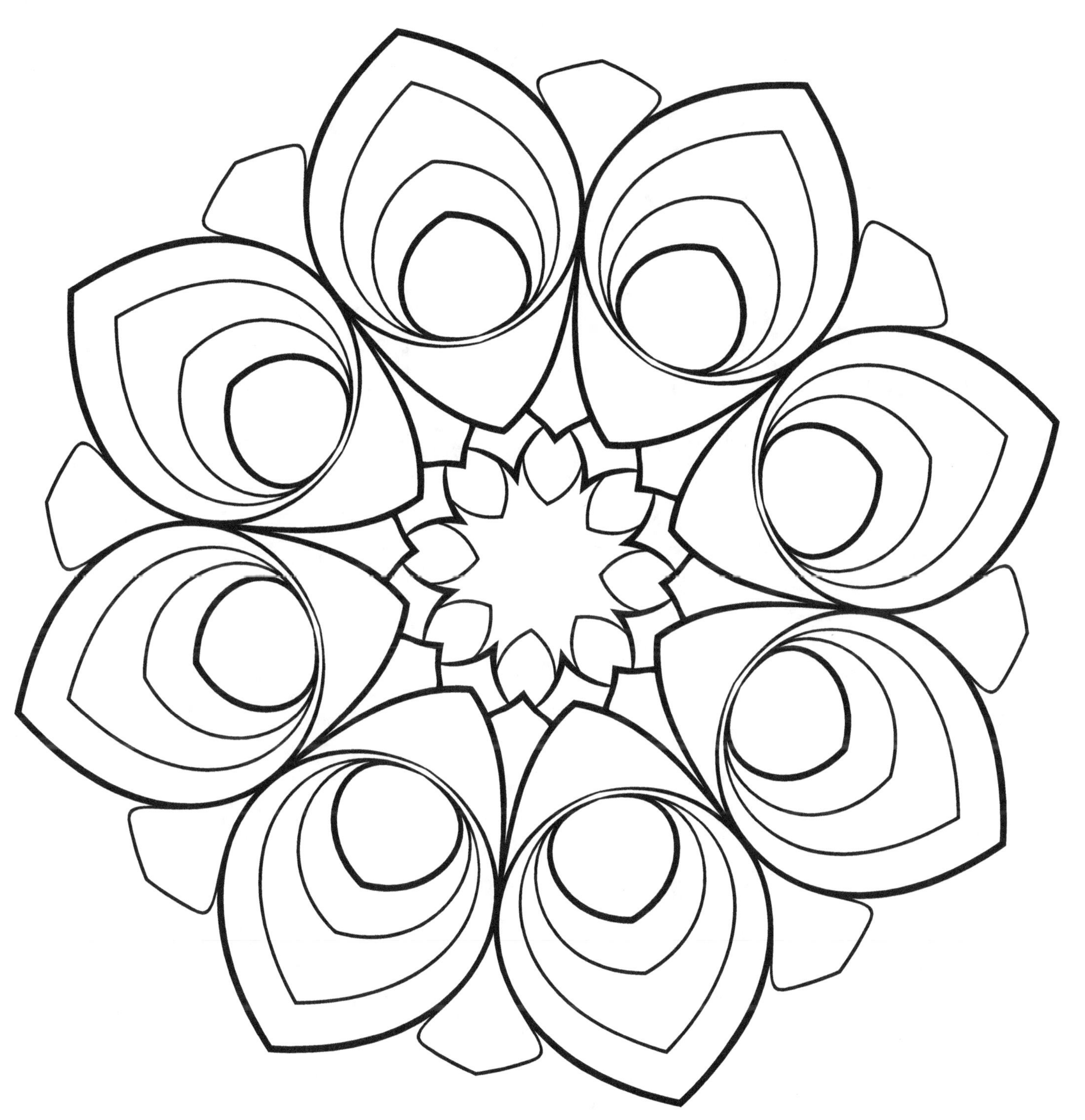

COLORING BOOK

by Little Mary

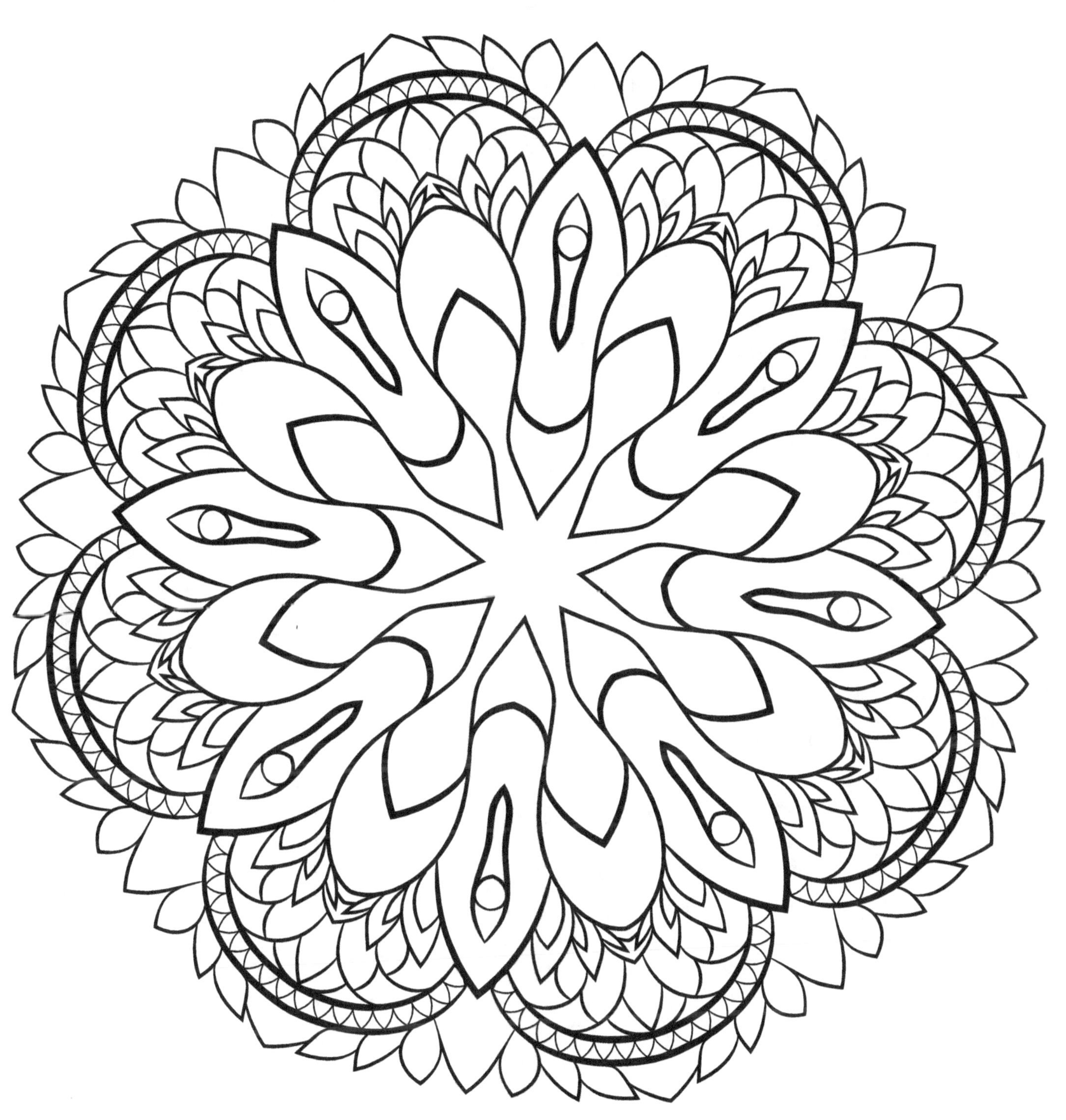

COLORING BOOK

by Little Mary

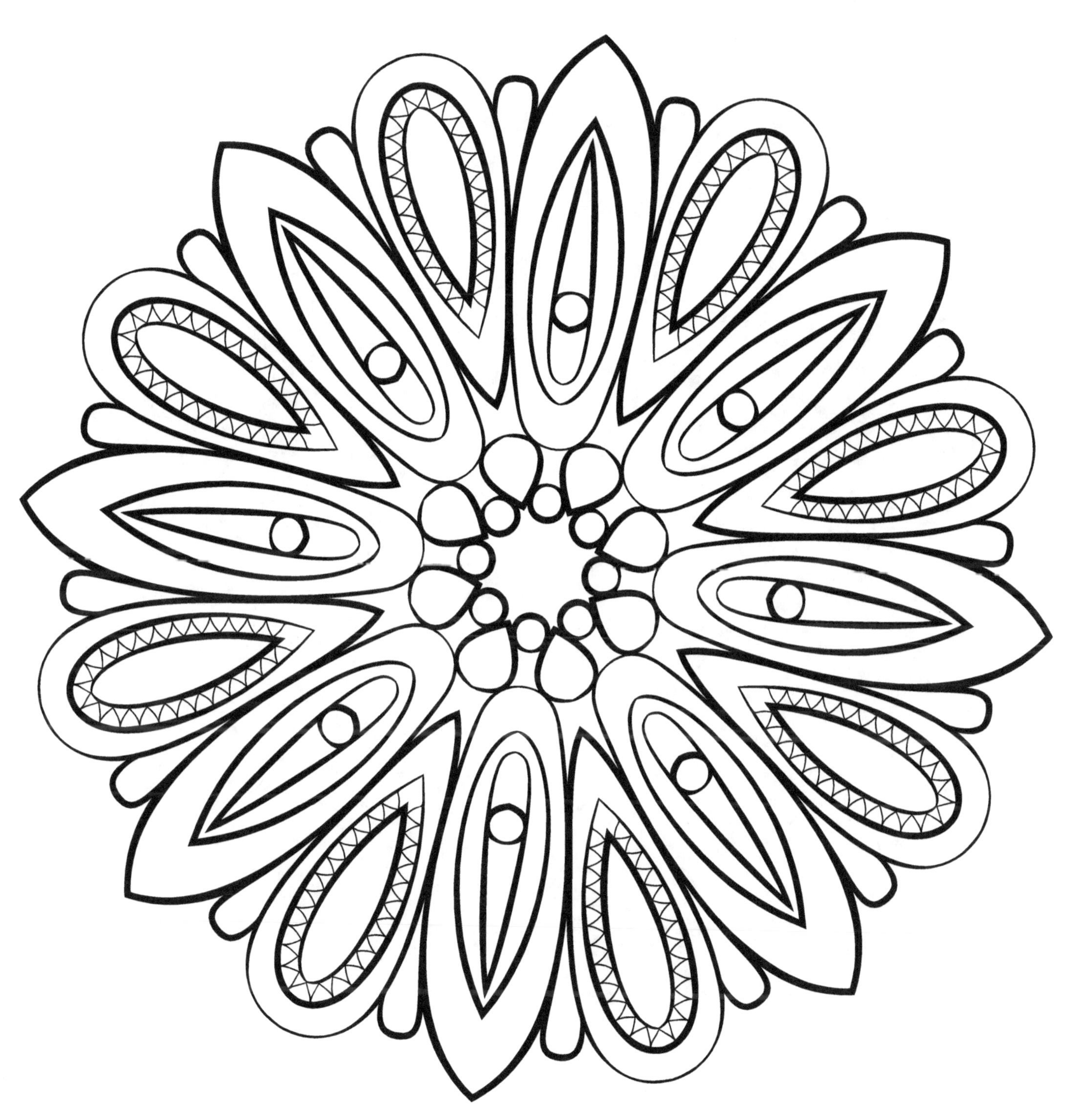

COLORING BOOK

by Little Mary

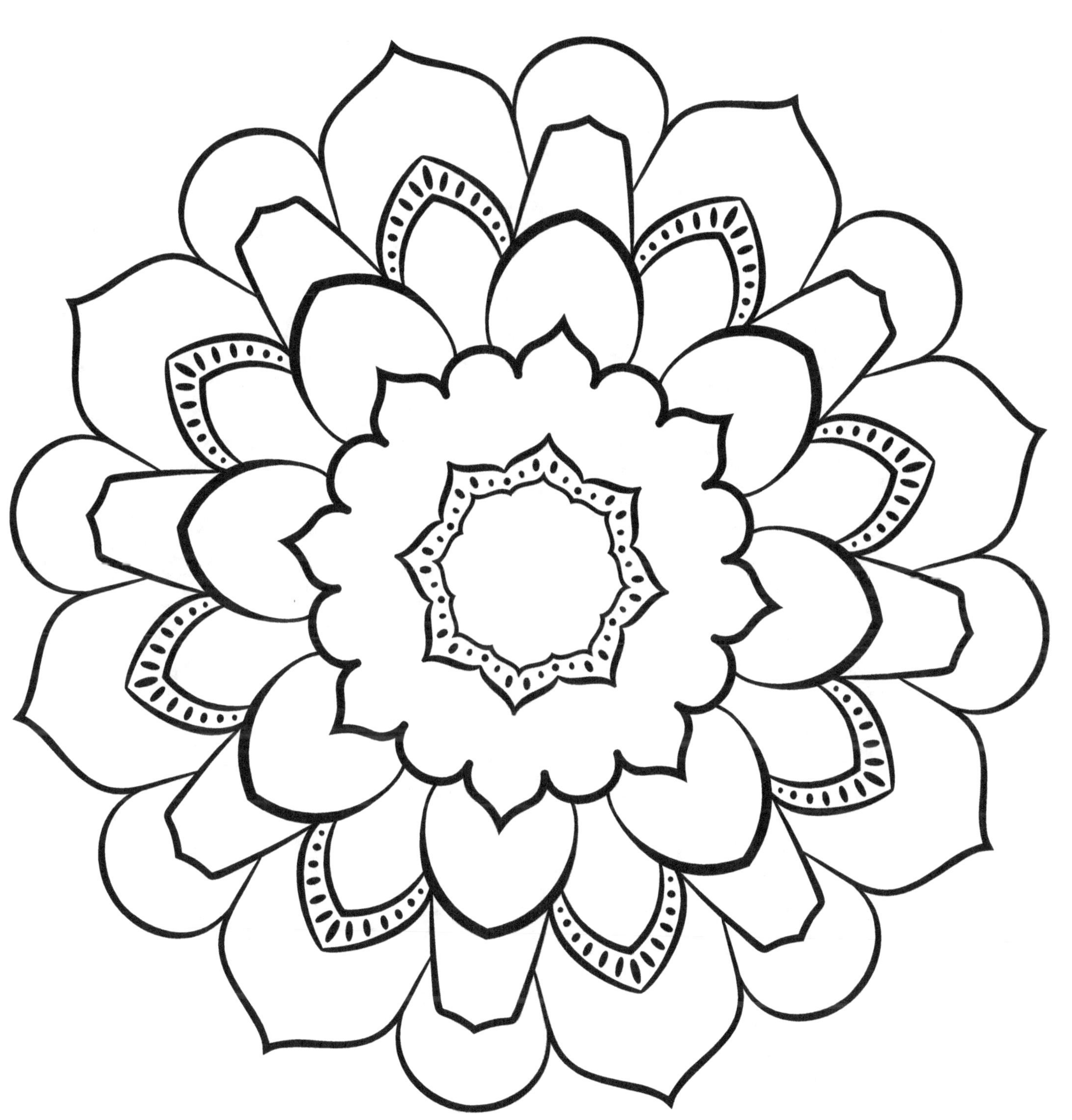

COLORING BOOK

by Little Mary

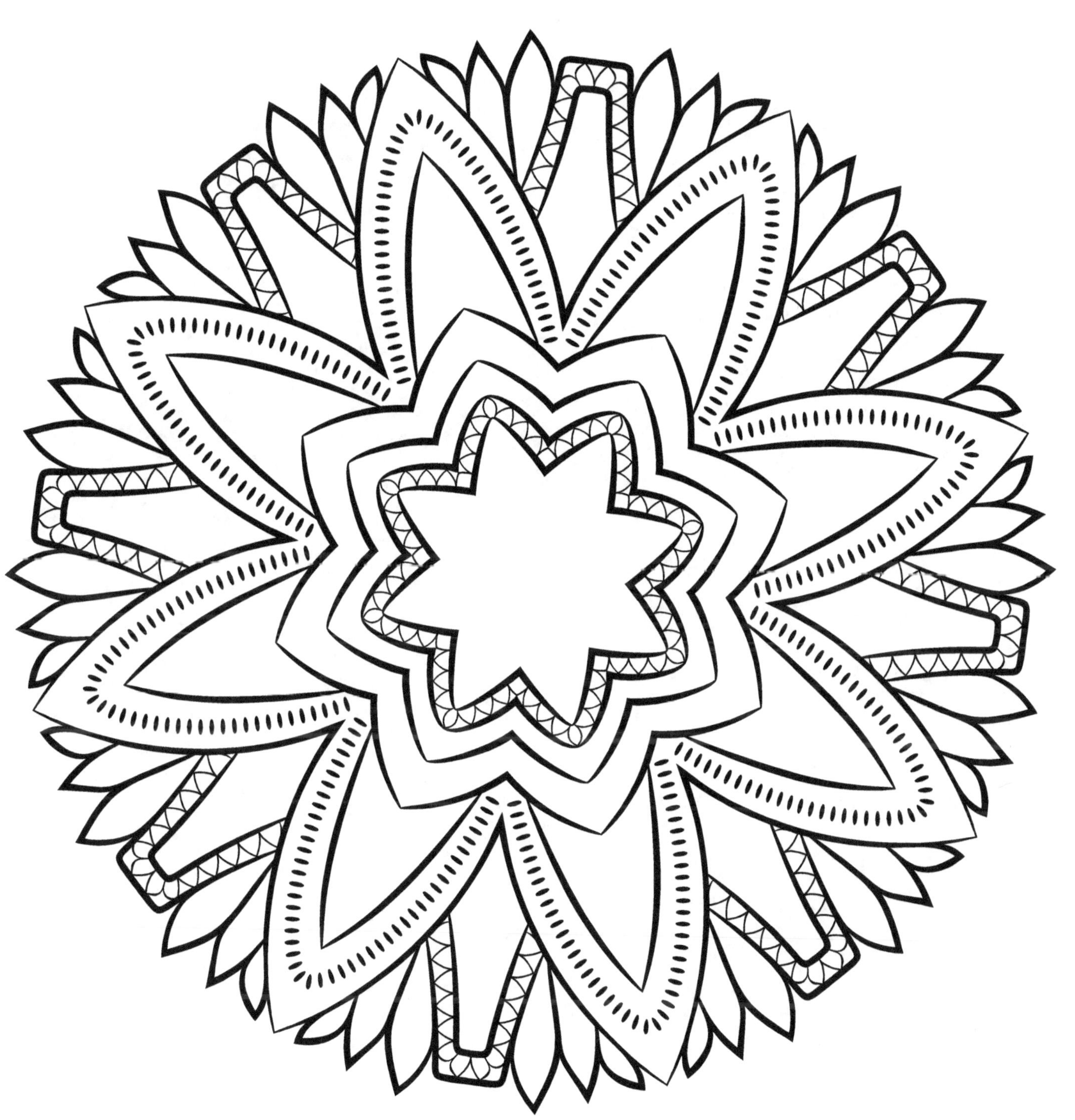

COLORING BOOK

by Little Mary

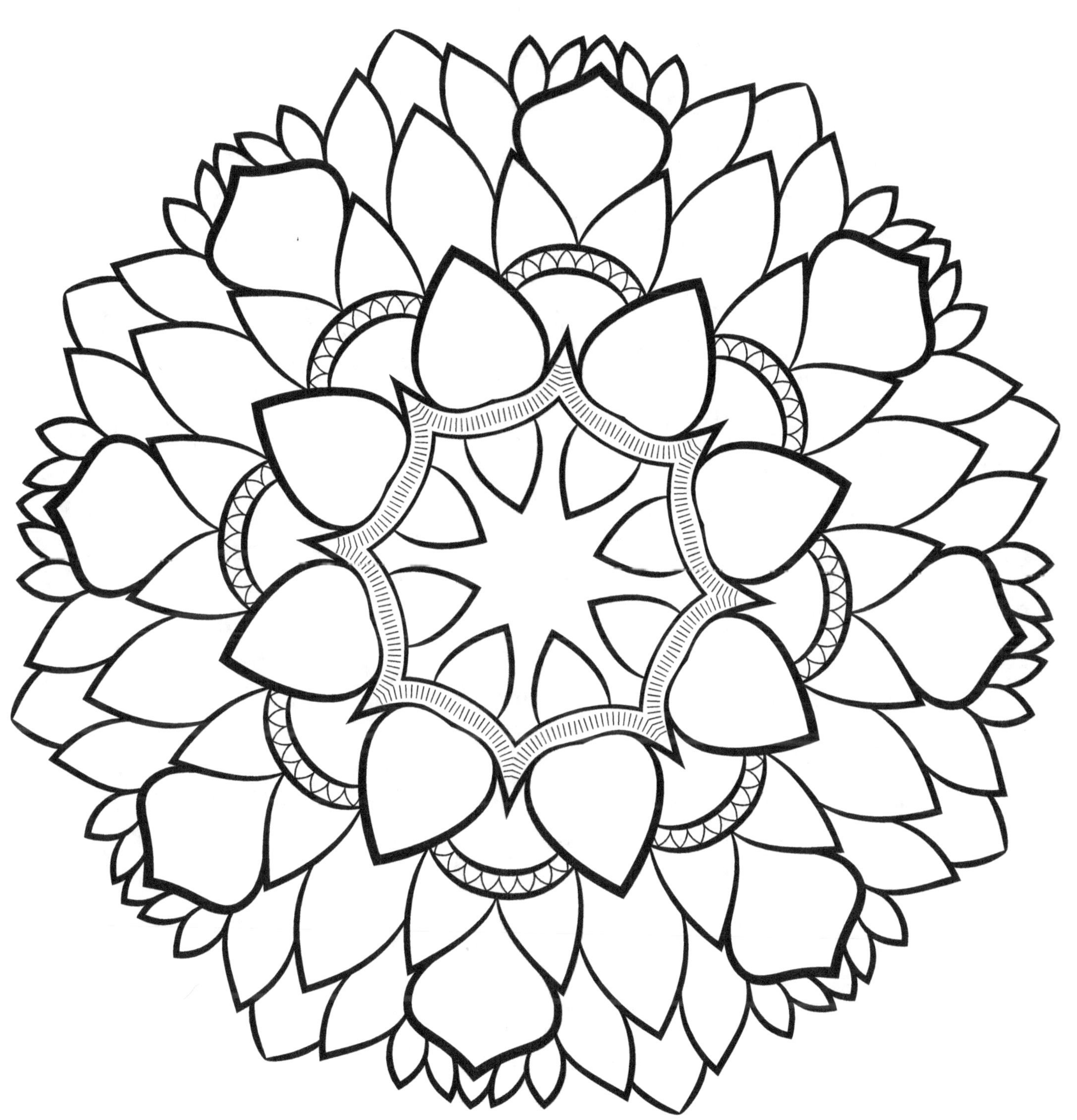

COLORING BOOK

by Little Mary

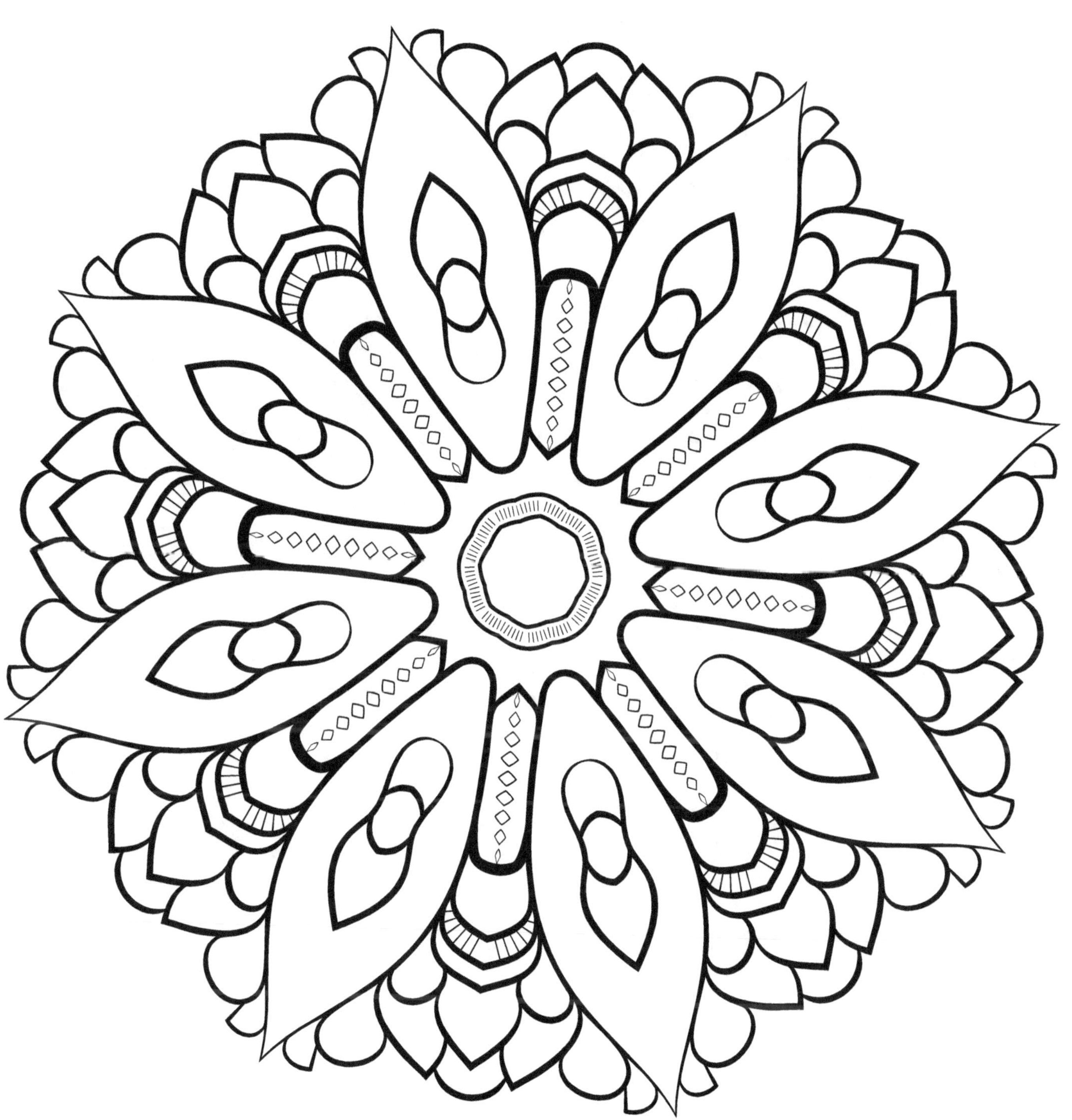

COLORING BOOK

by Little Mary

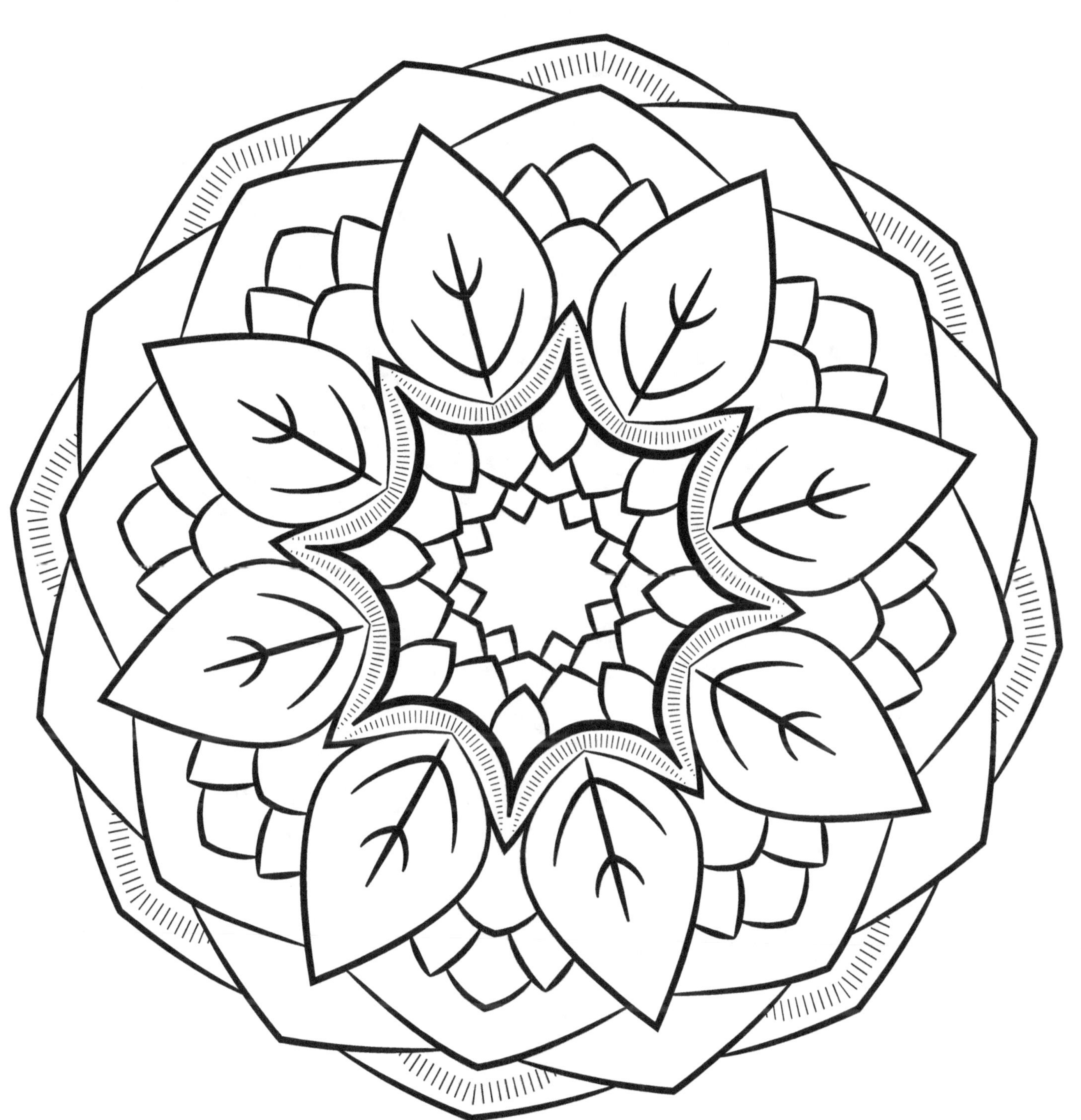

COLORING BOOK

by Little Mary

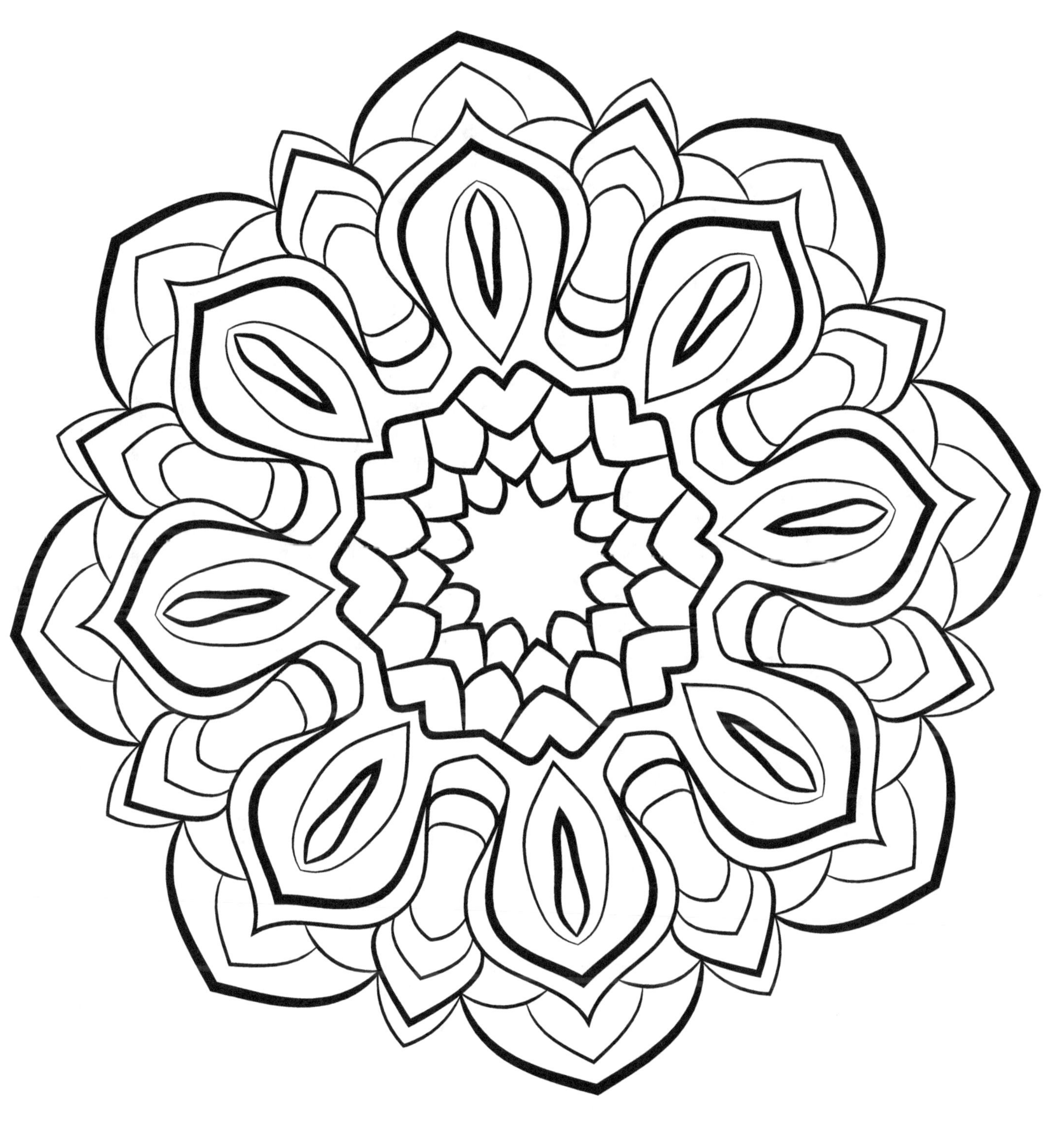

COLORING BOOK

by Little Mary

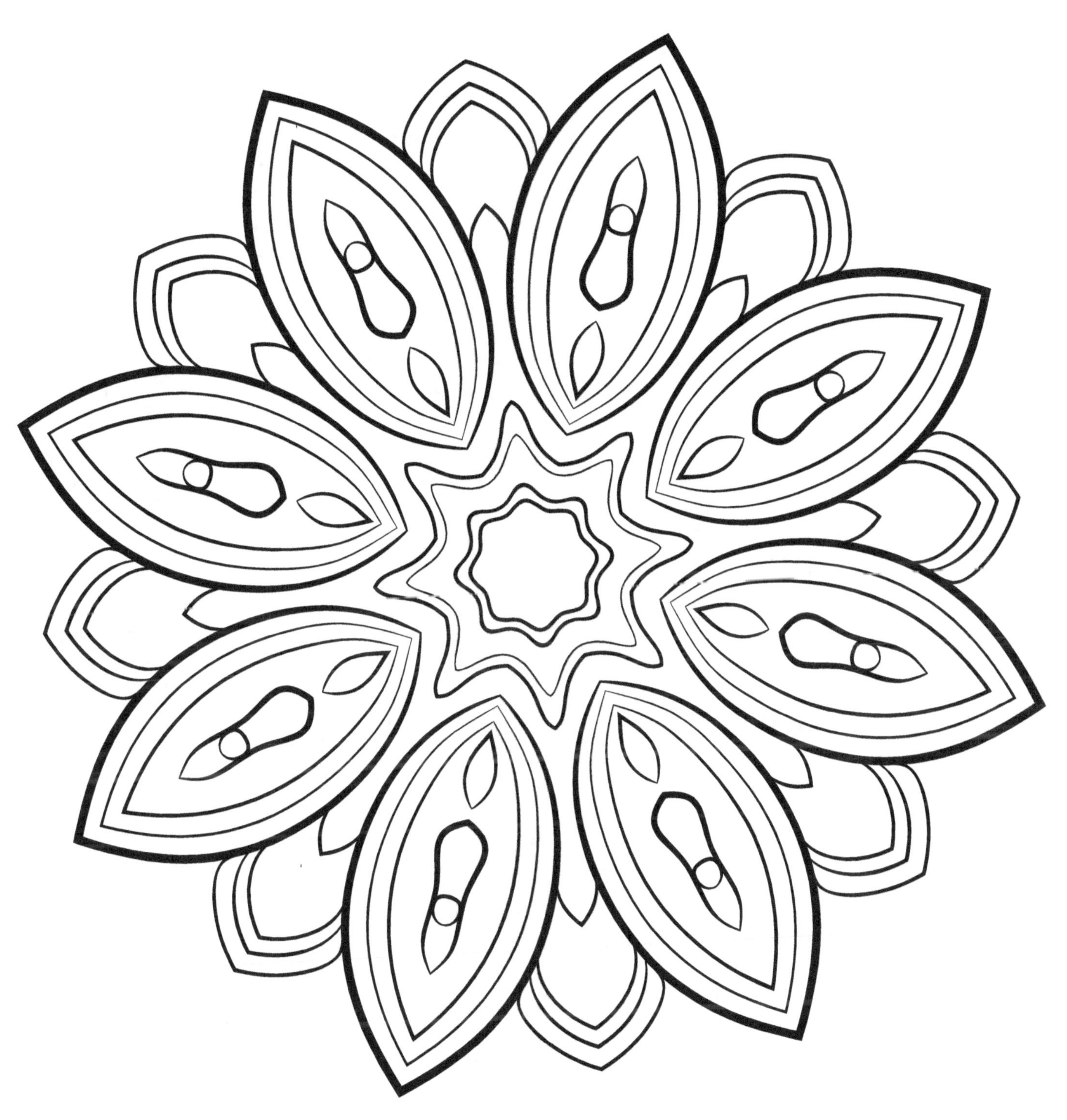

COLORING BOOK

by Little Mary

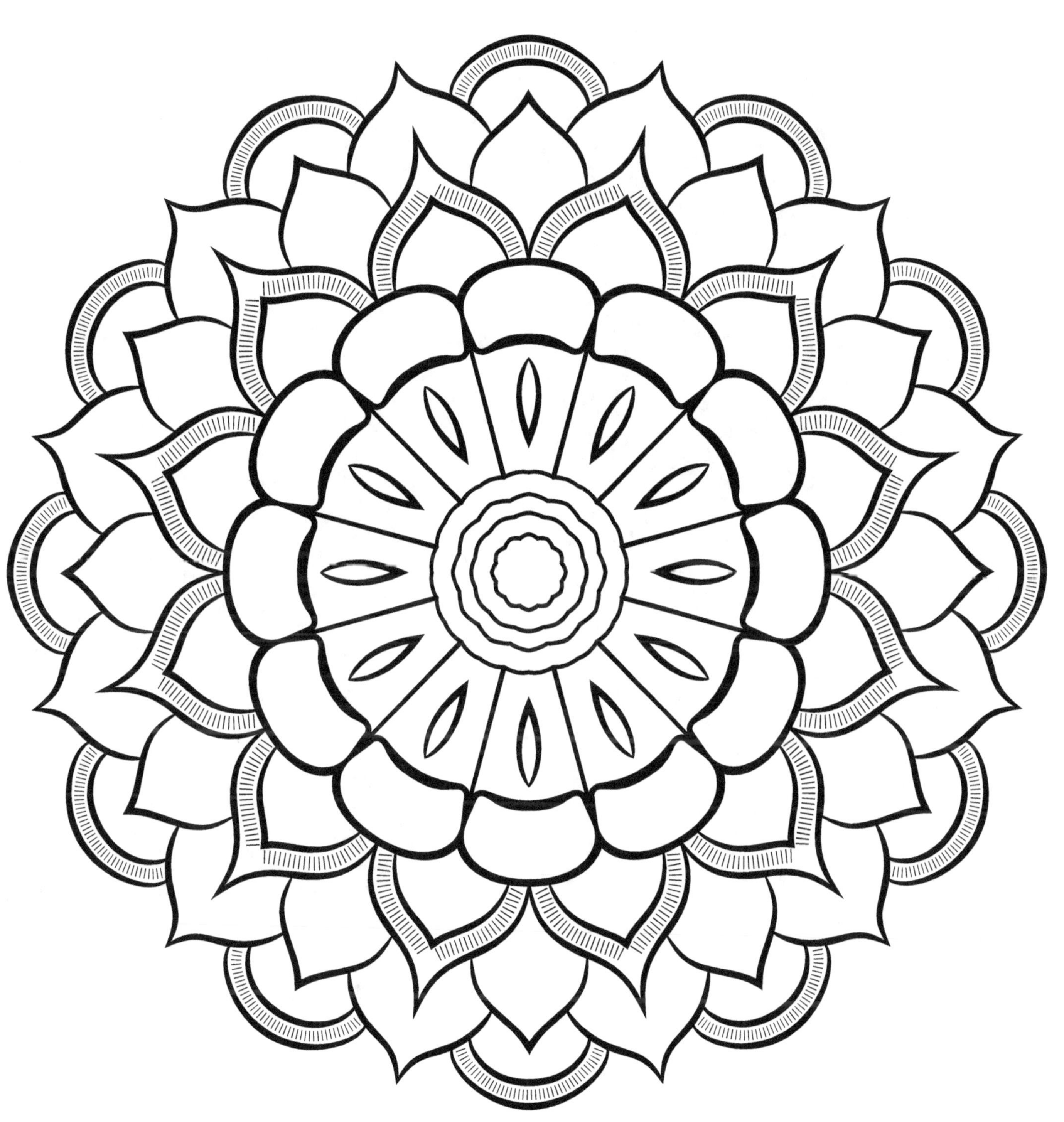

COLORING BOOK

by Little Mary

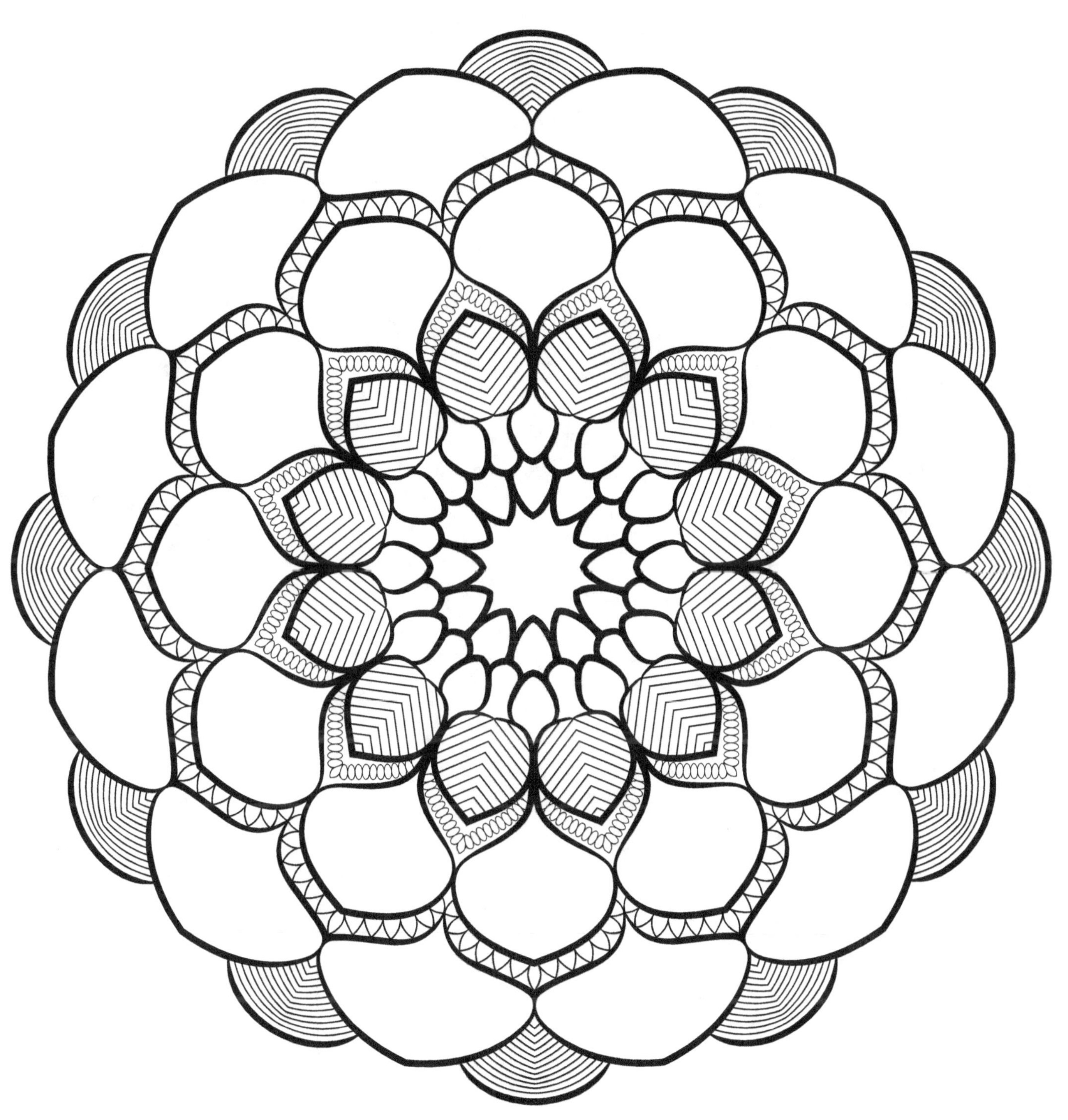

COLORING BOOK

by Little Mary

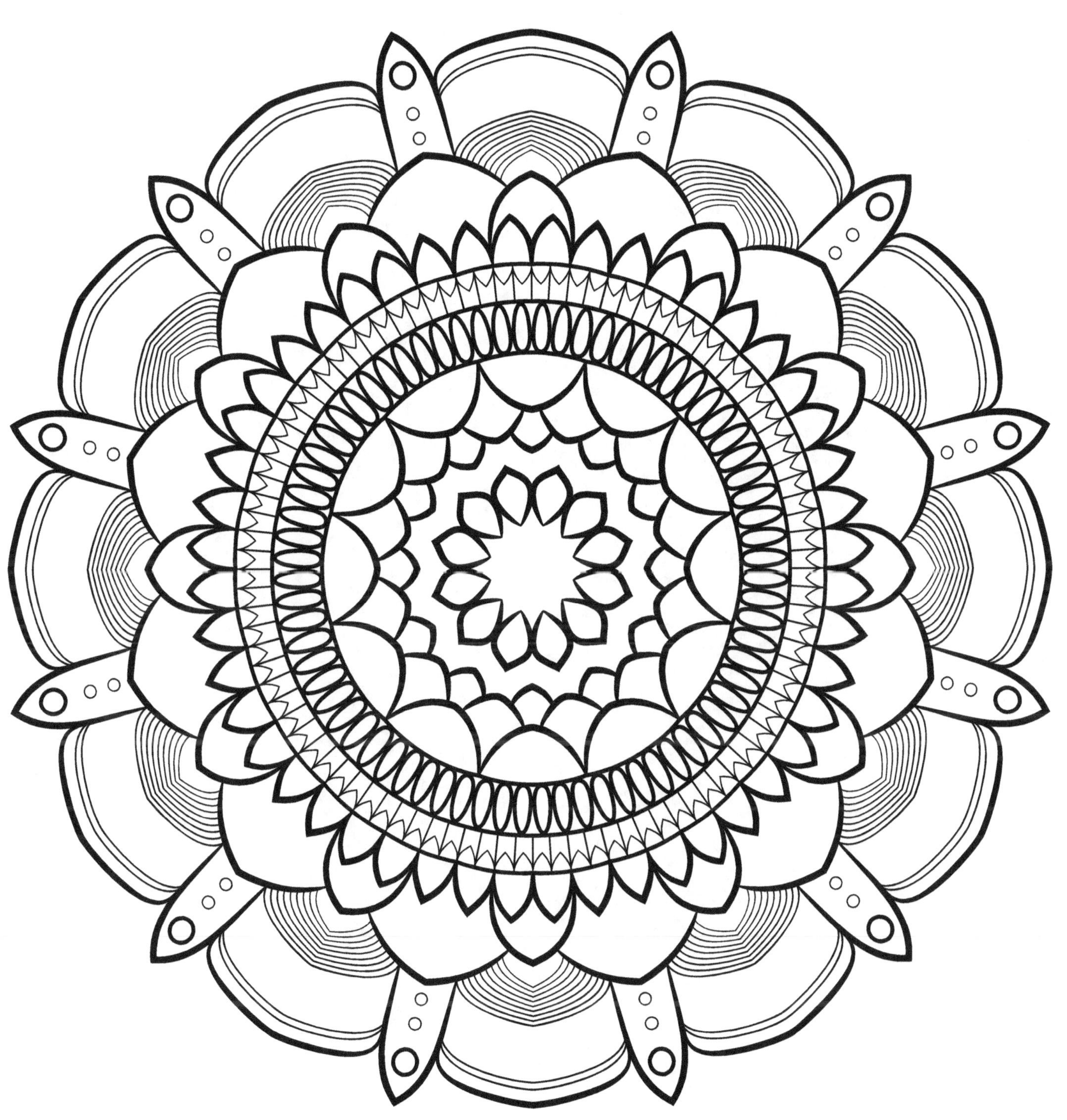

COLORING BOOK

by Little Mary

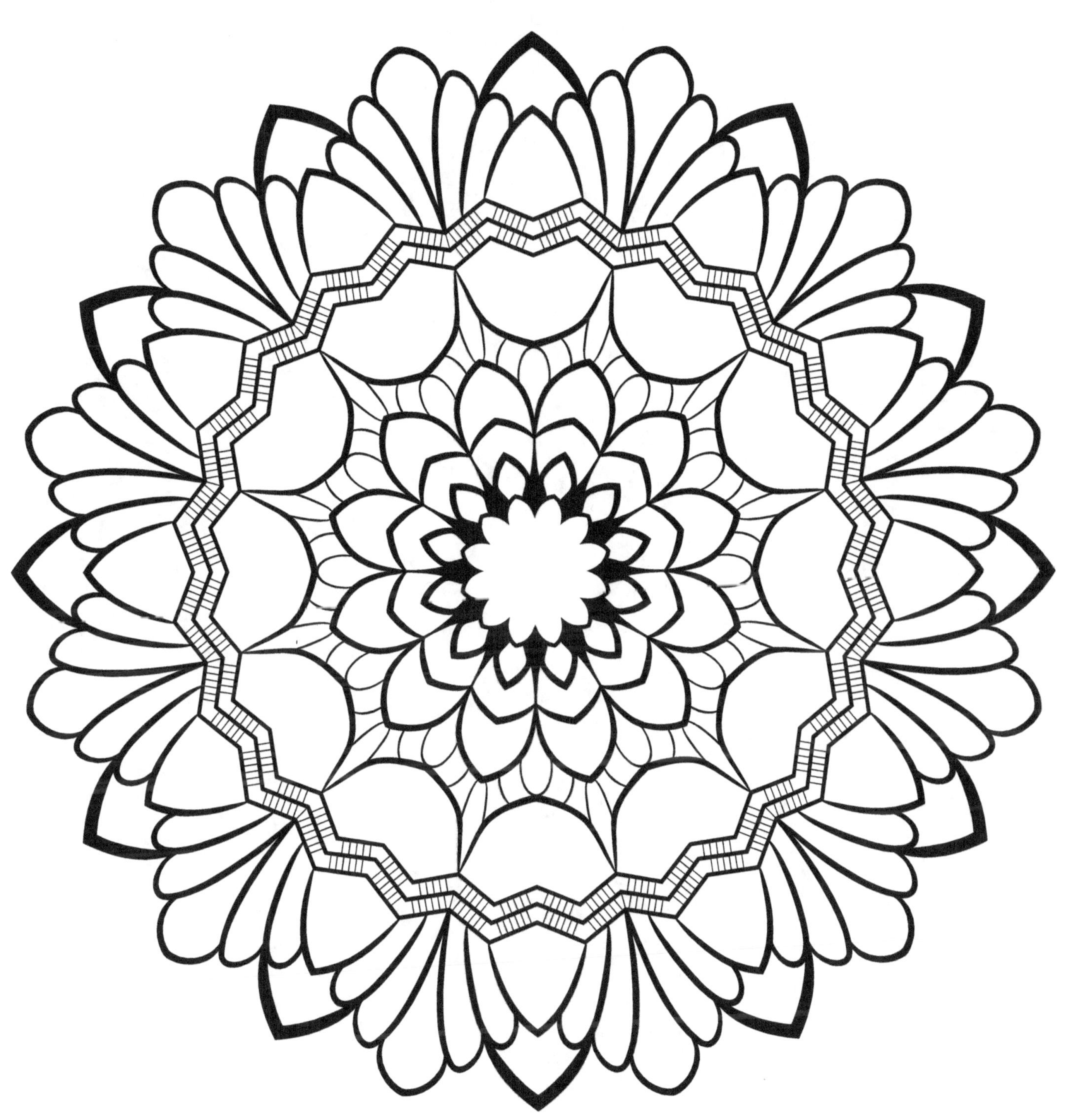

COLORING BOOK

by Little Mary

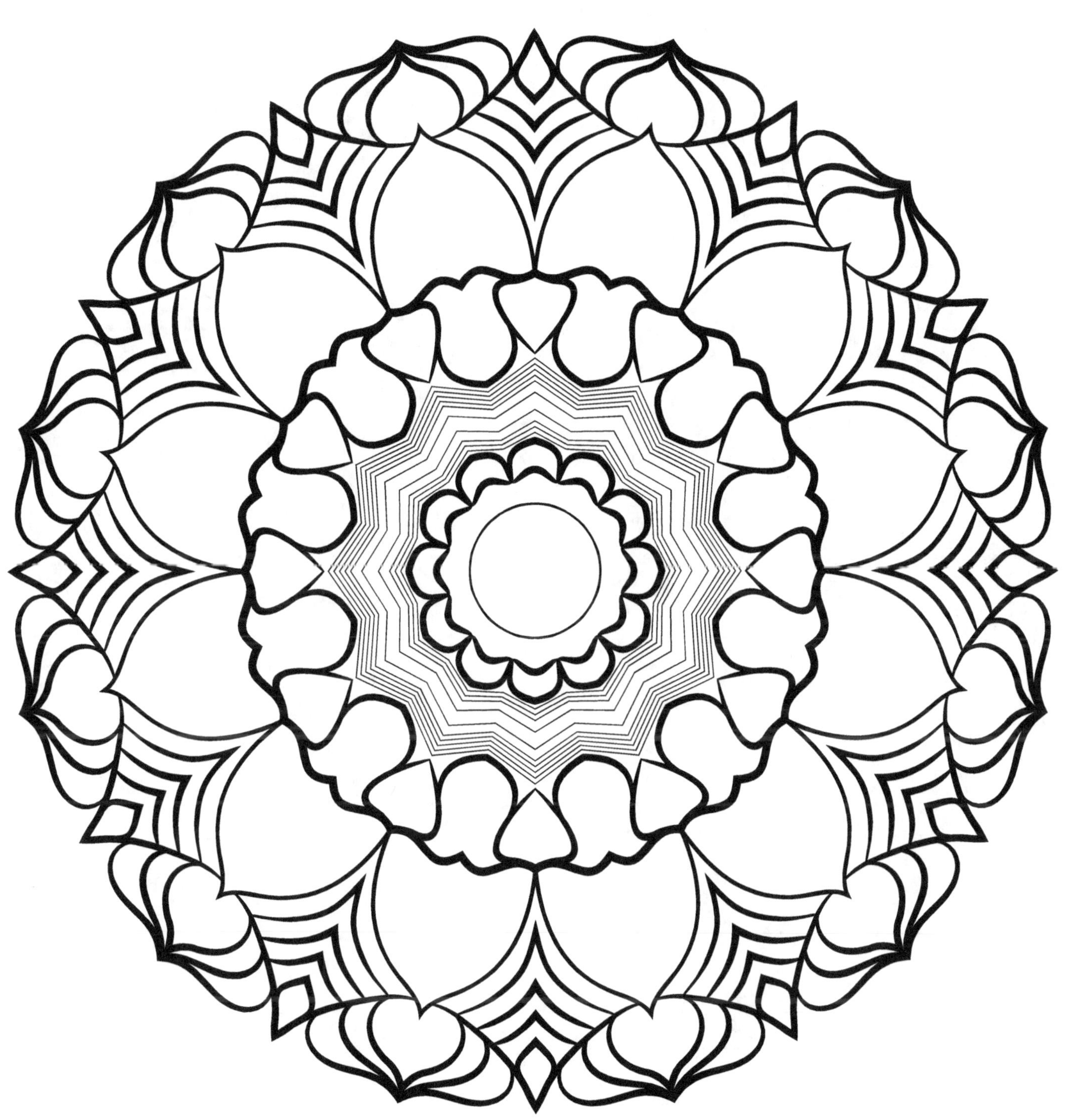

COLORING BOOK

by Little Mary

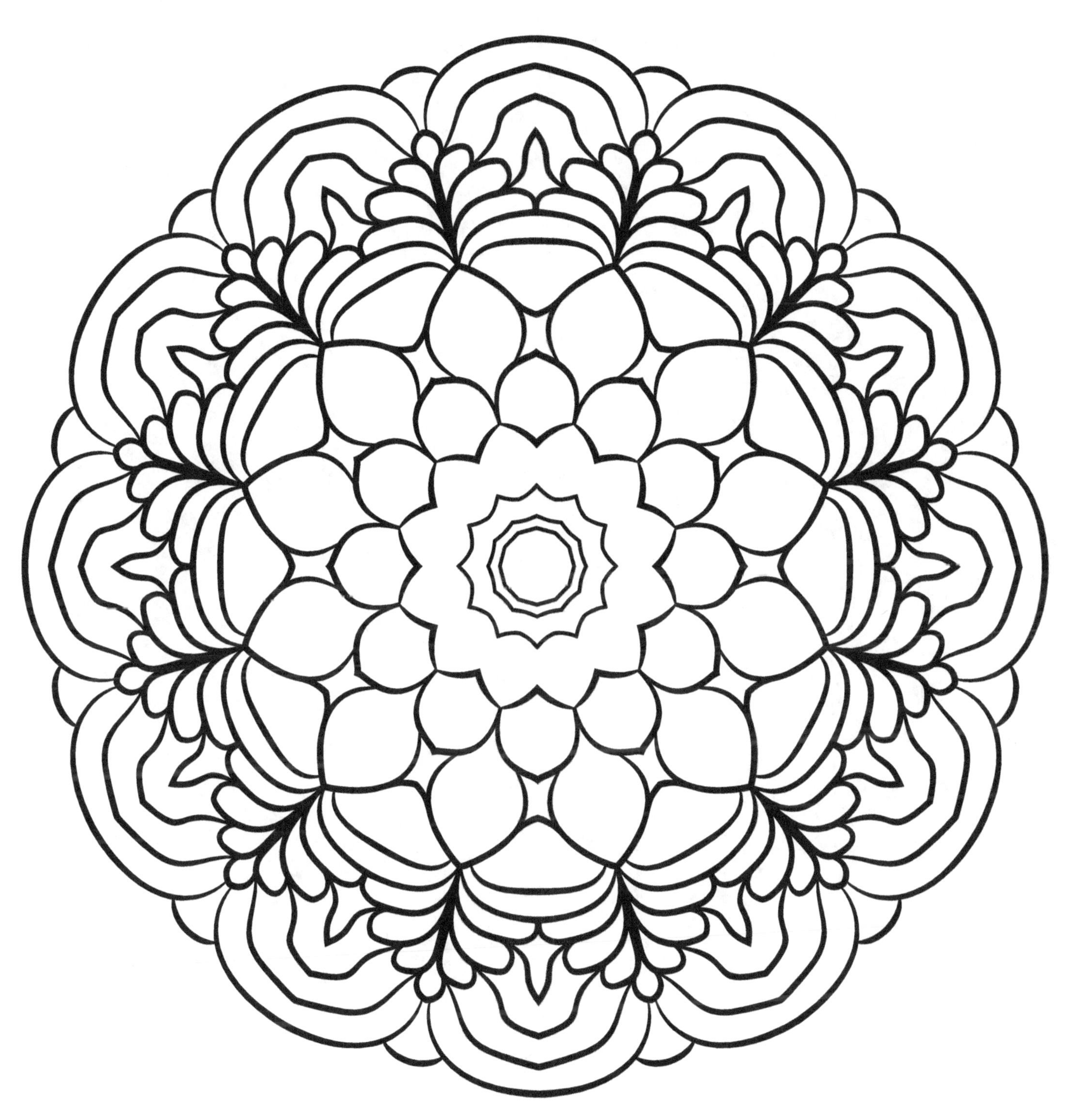

COLORING BOOK

by Little Mary

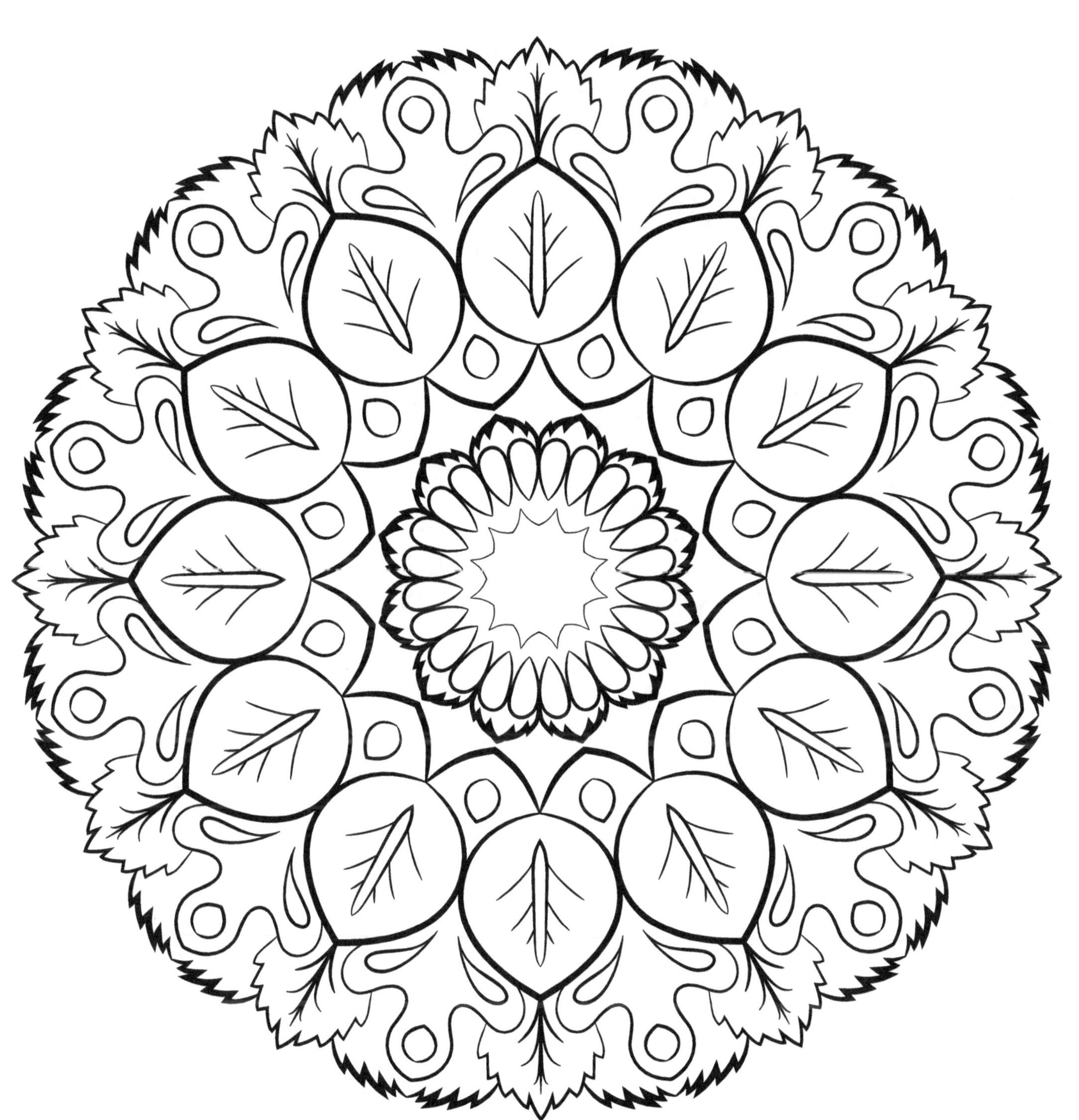

COLORING BOOK

by Little Mary

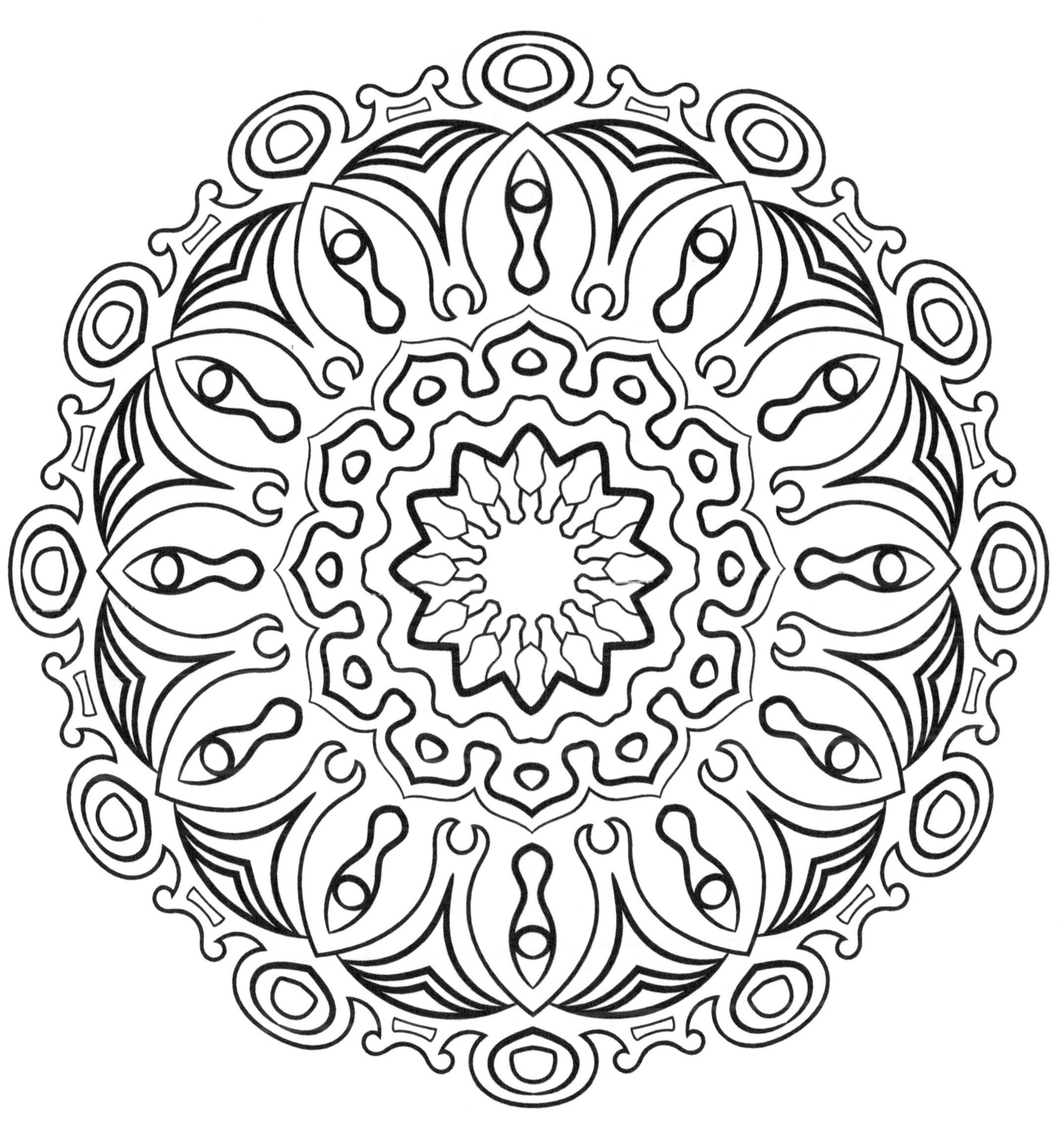

COLORING BOOK

by Little Mary

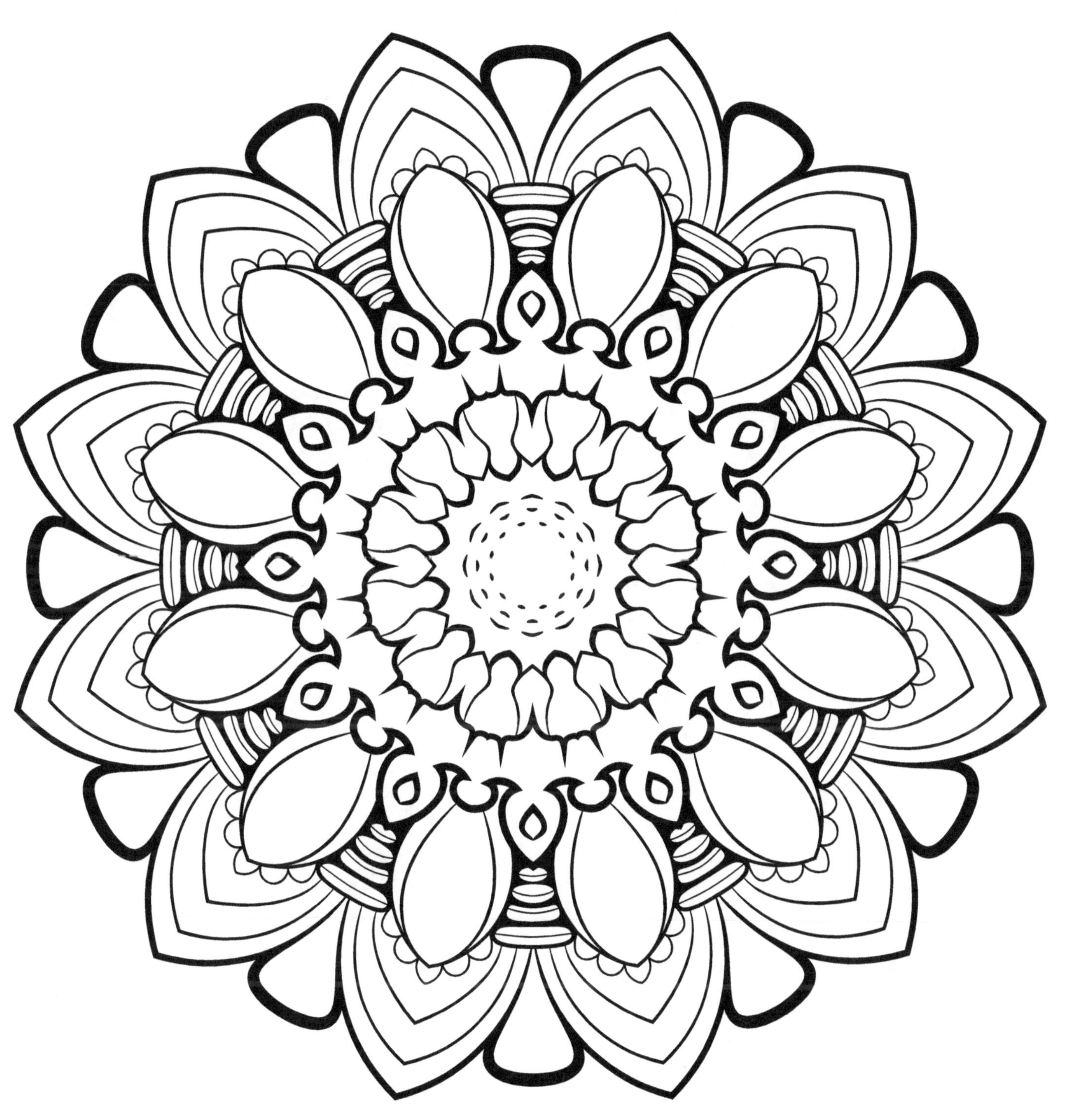

COLORING BOOK

by Little Mary

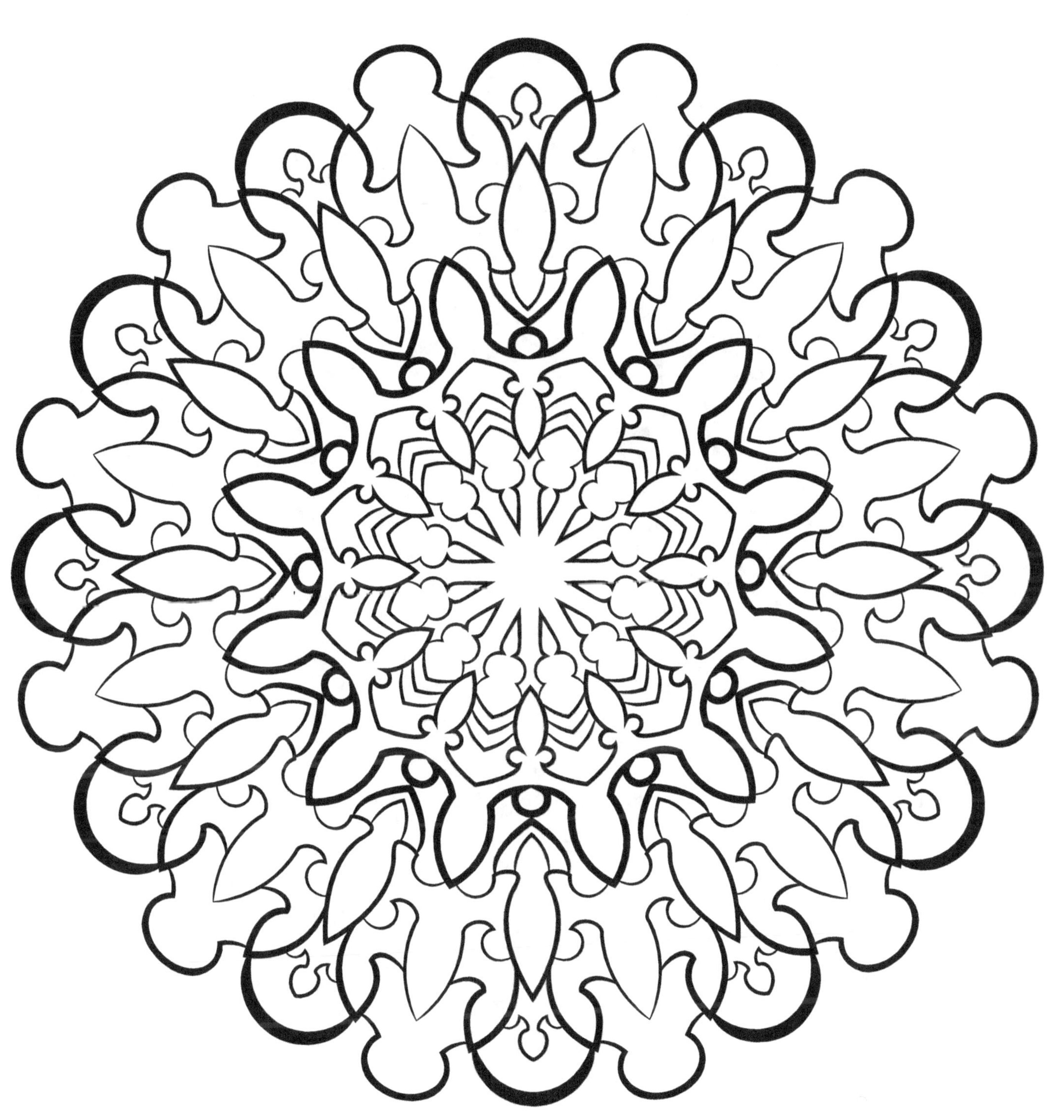

COLORING BOOK

by Little Mary

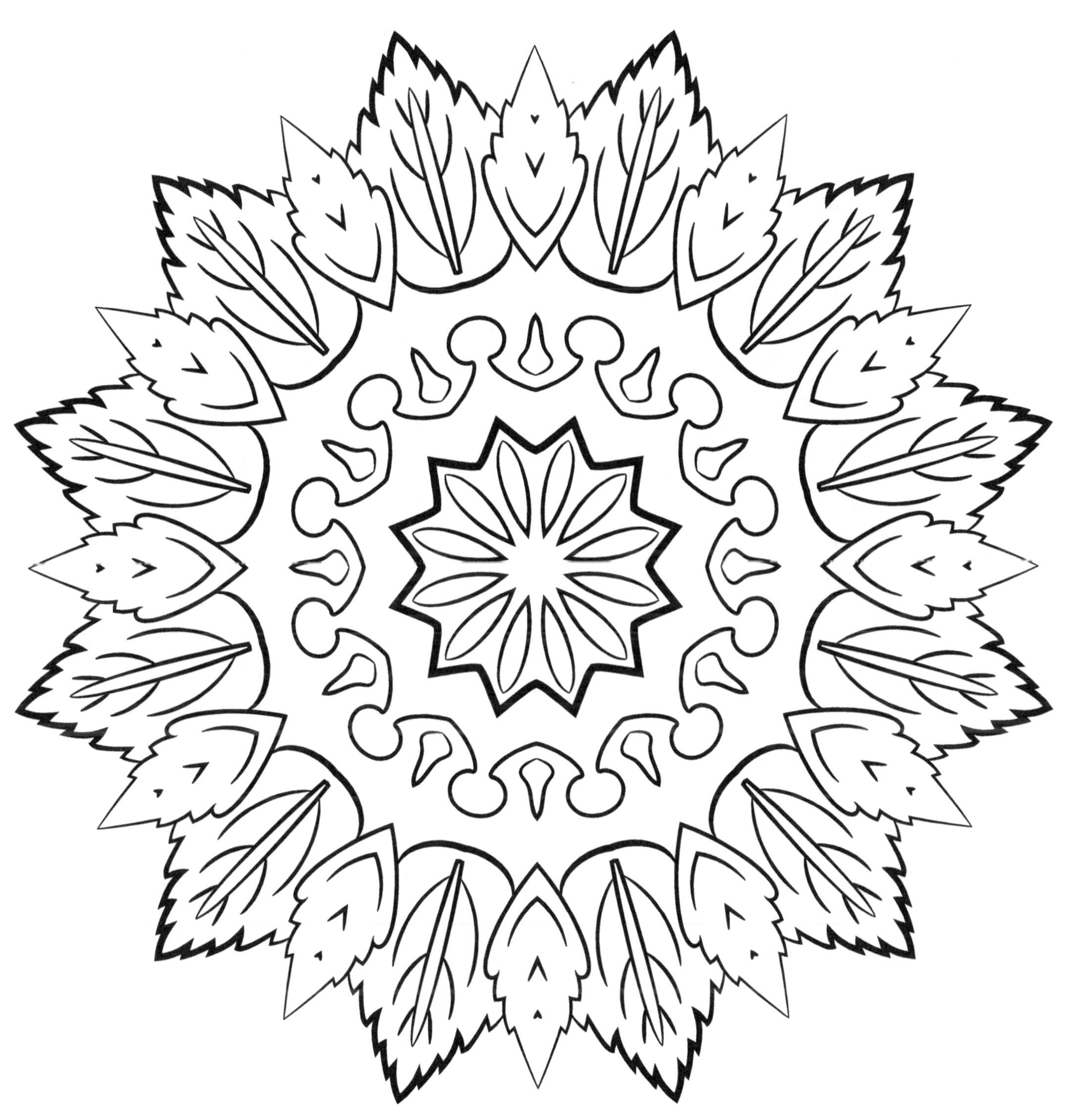

COLORING BOOK

by Little Mary

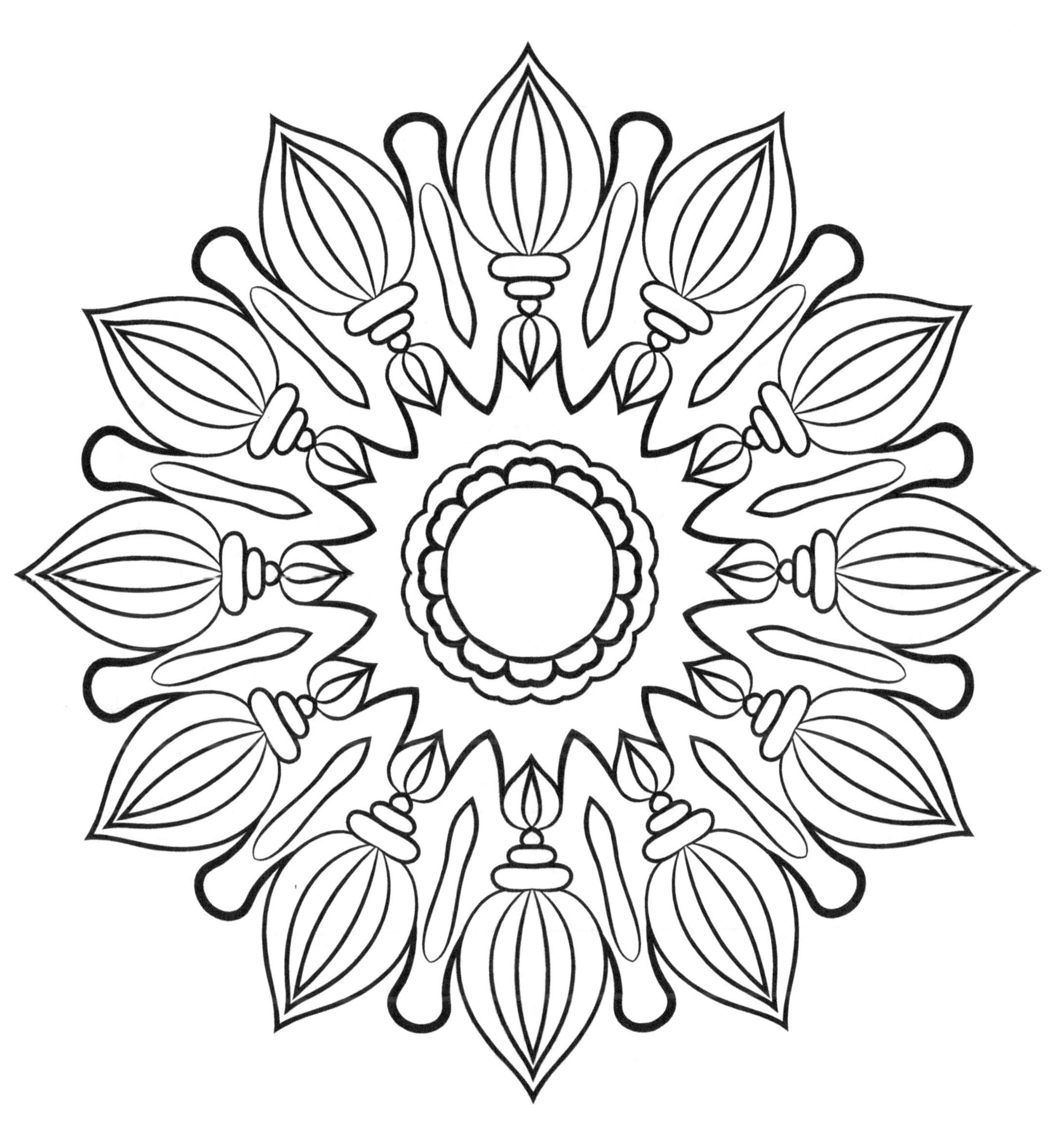

COLORING BOOK

by Little Mary

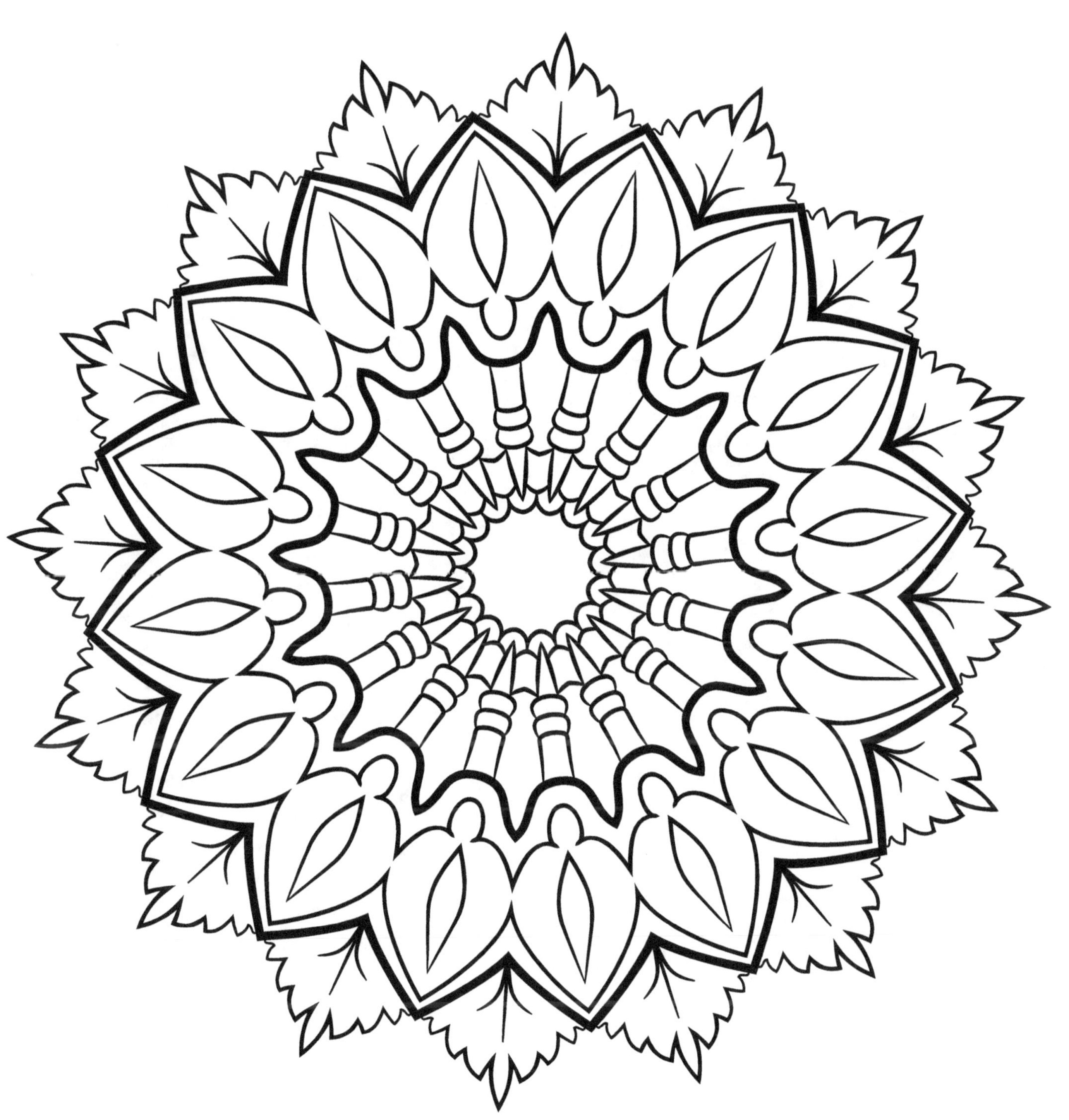

COLORING BOOK

by Little Mary

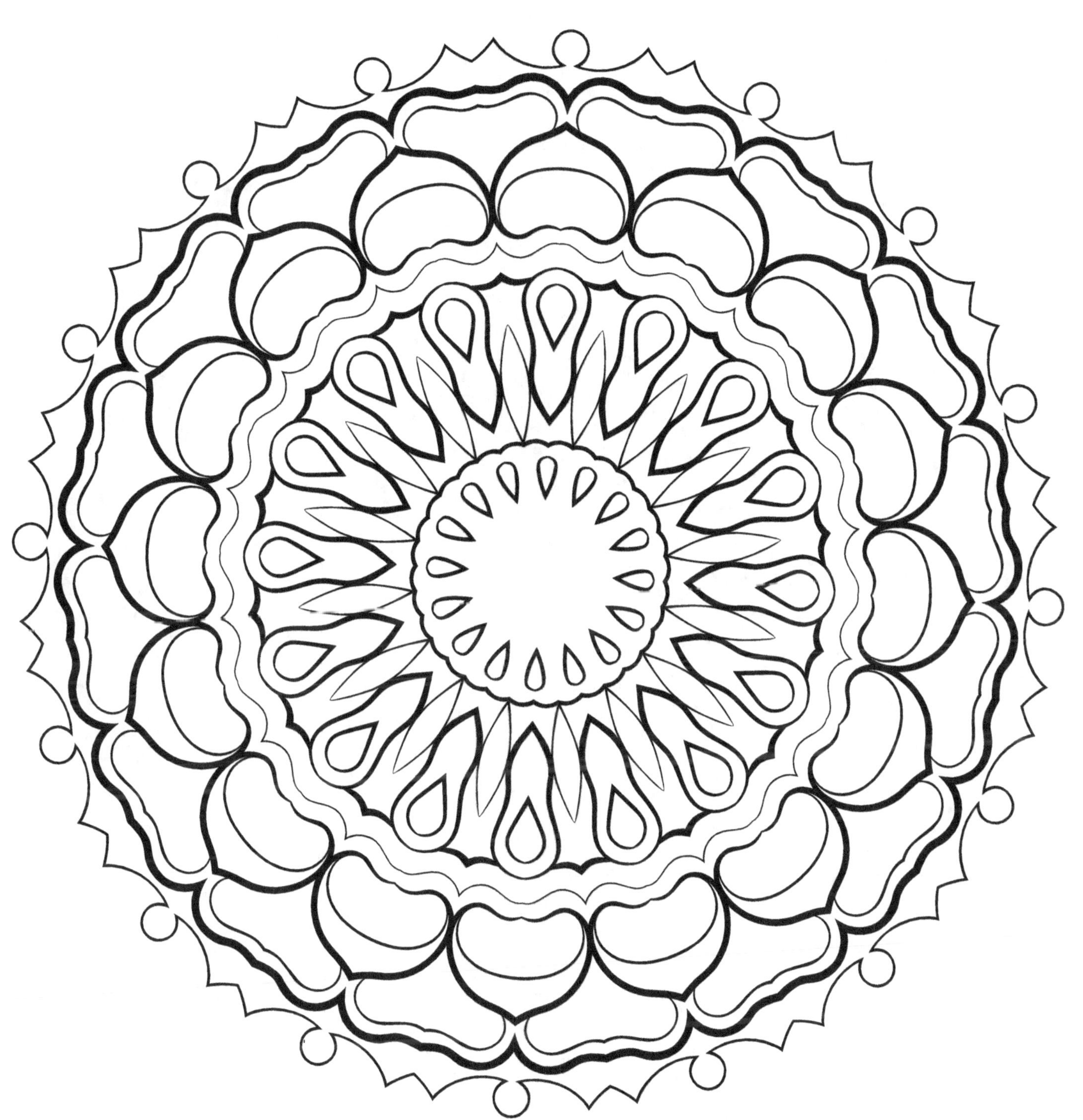

COLORING BOOK

by Little Mary

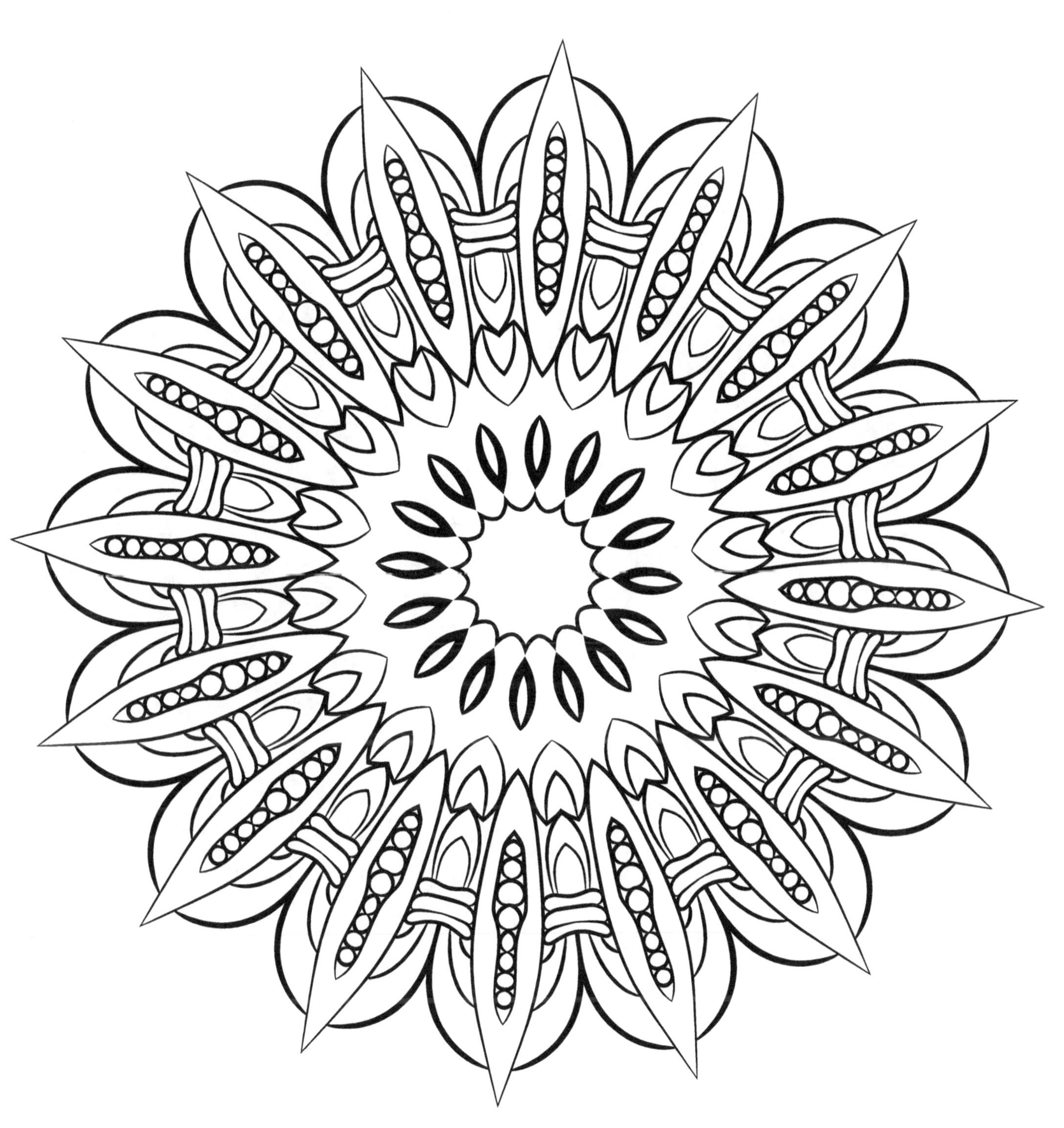

COLORING BOOK

by Little Mary

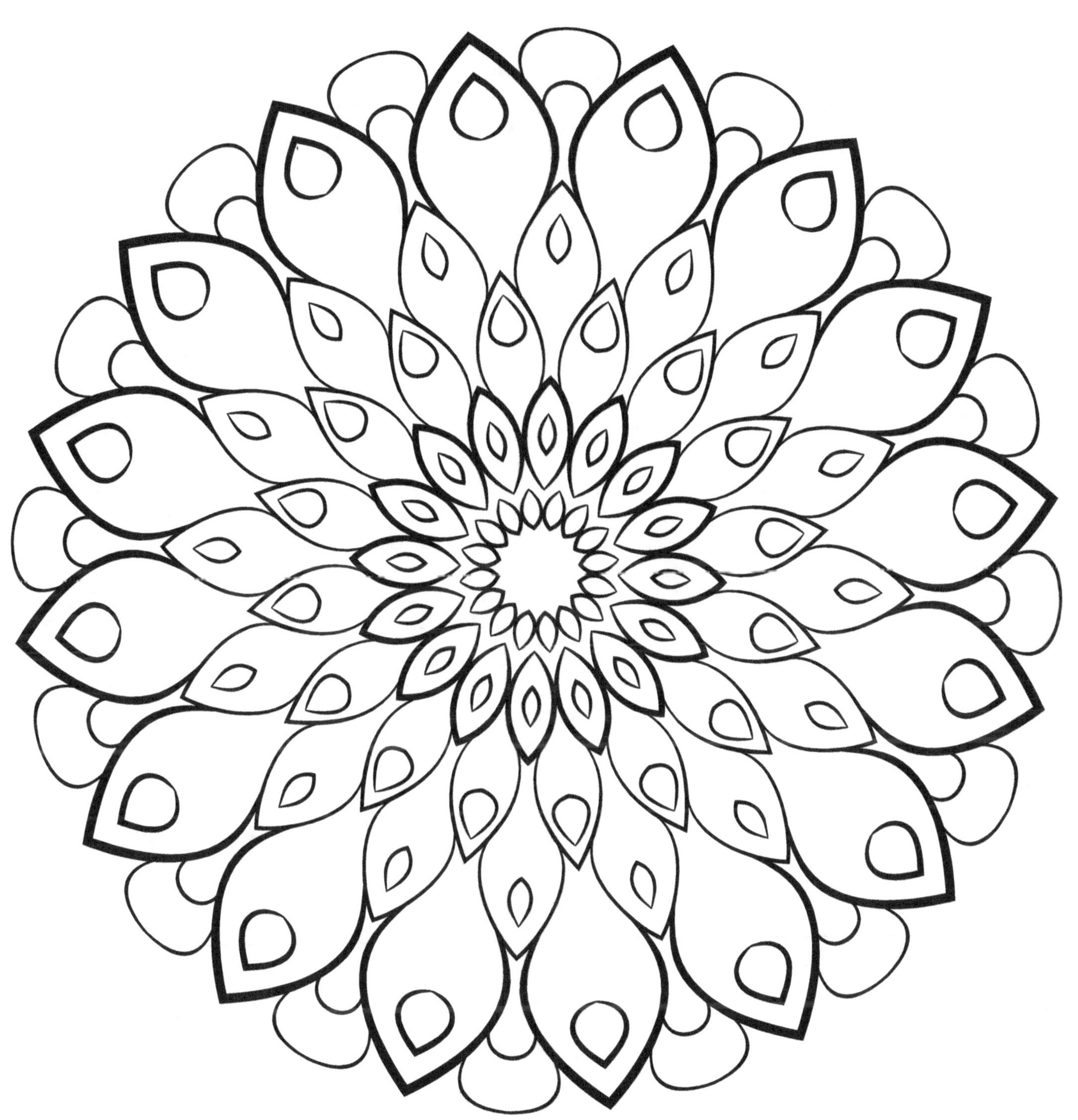

COLORING BOOK

by Little Mary

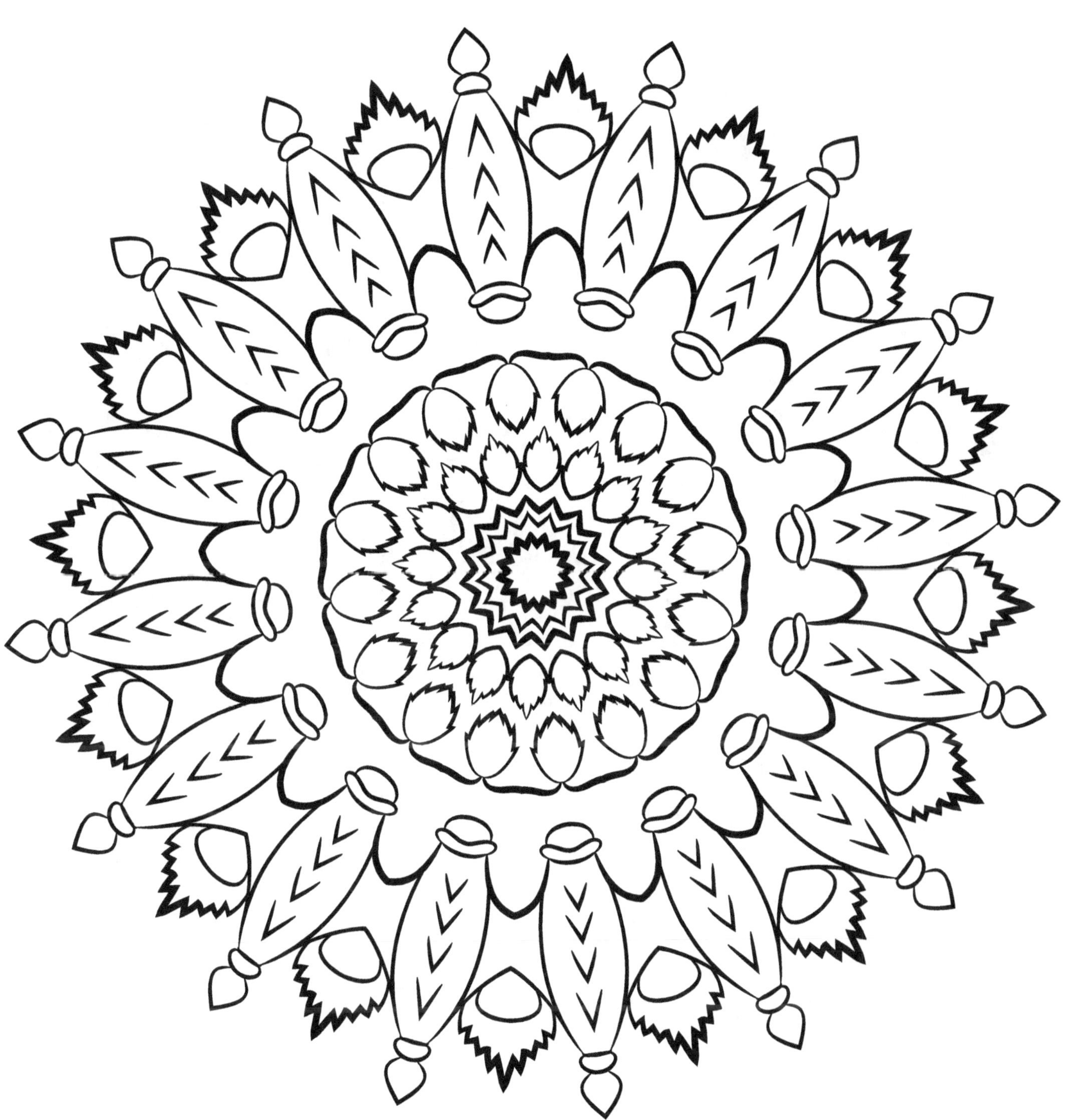

COLORING BOOK

by Little Mary

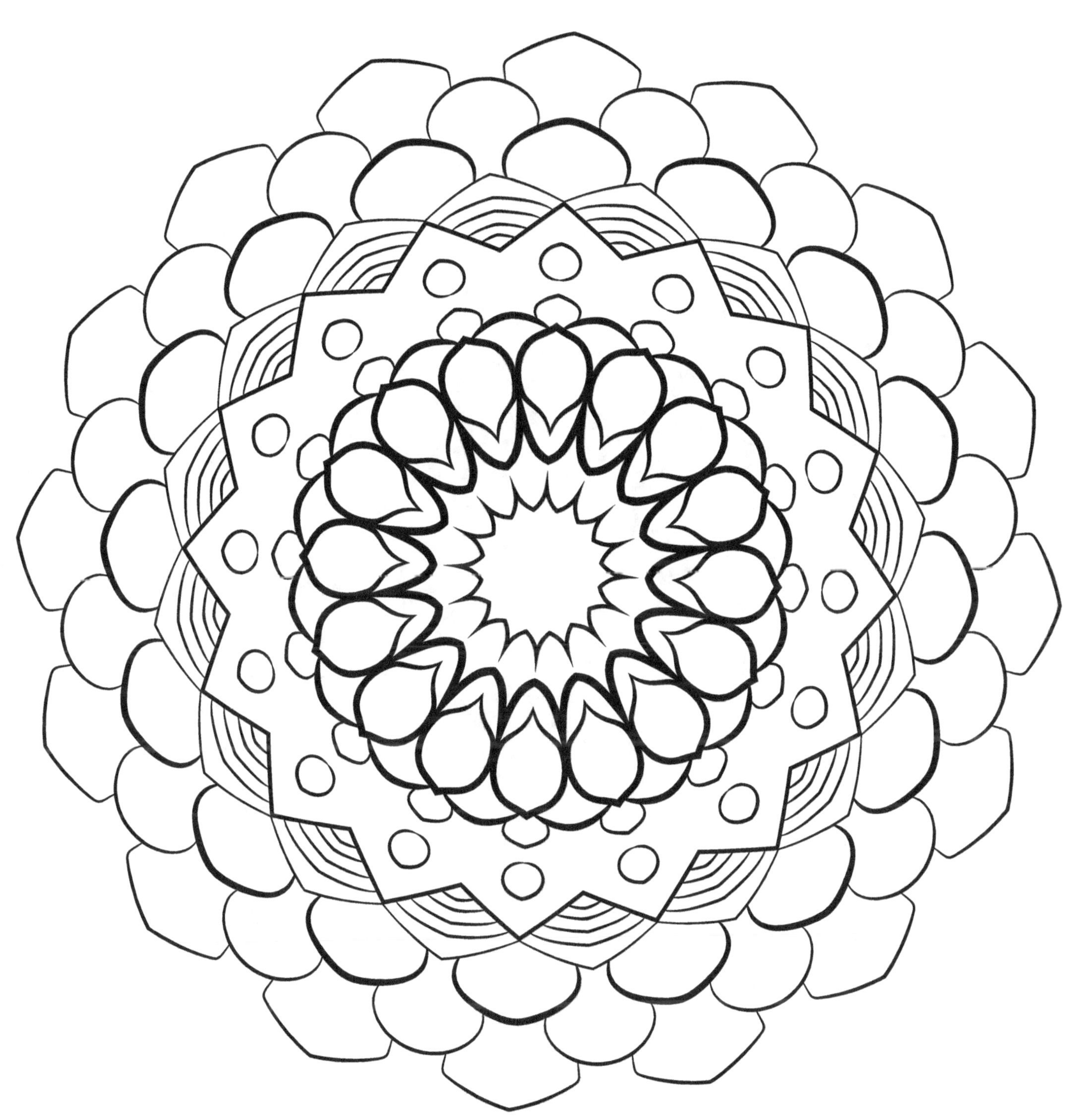

COLORING BOOK

by Little Mary

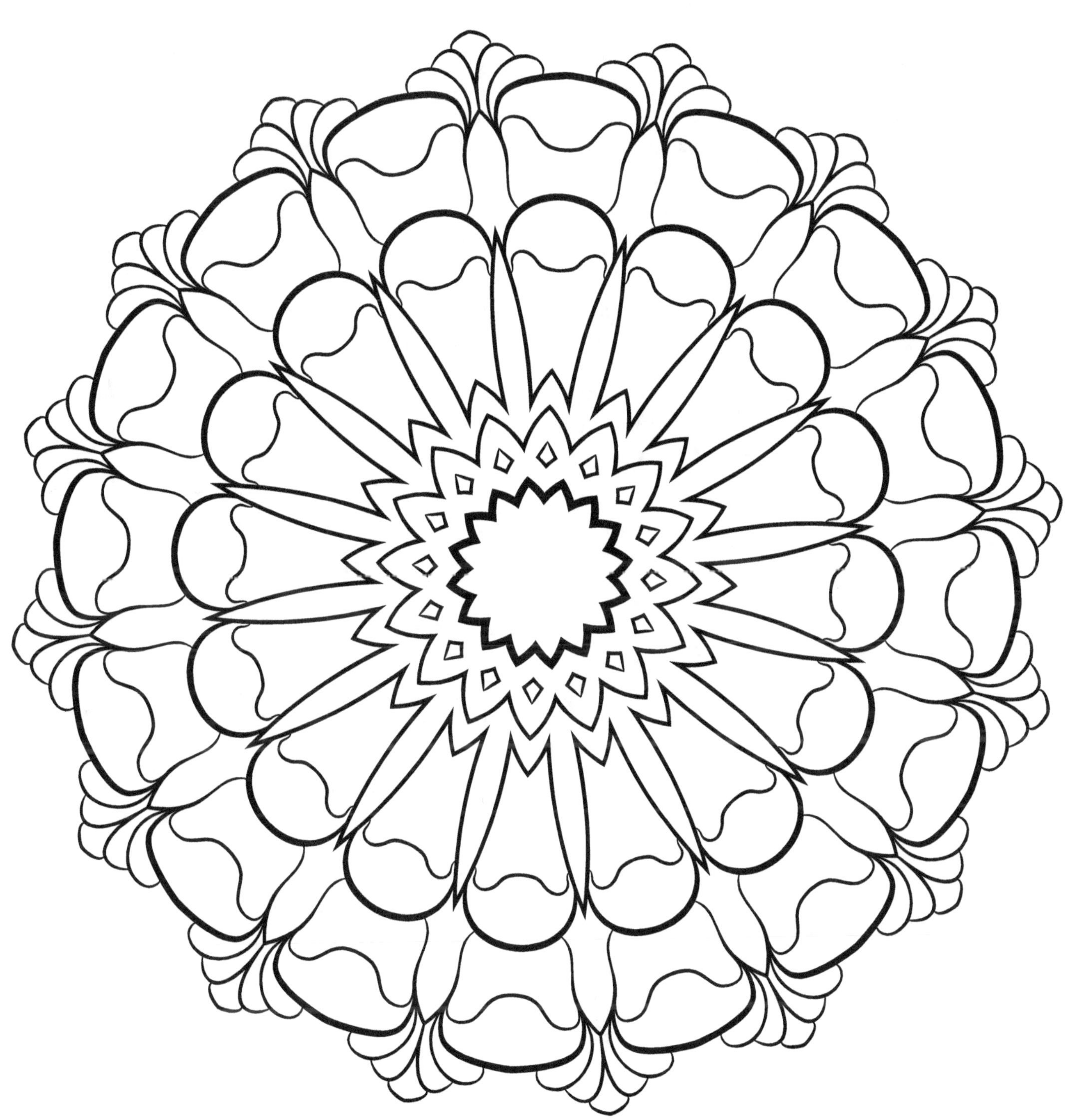

COLORING BOOK

by Little Mary

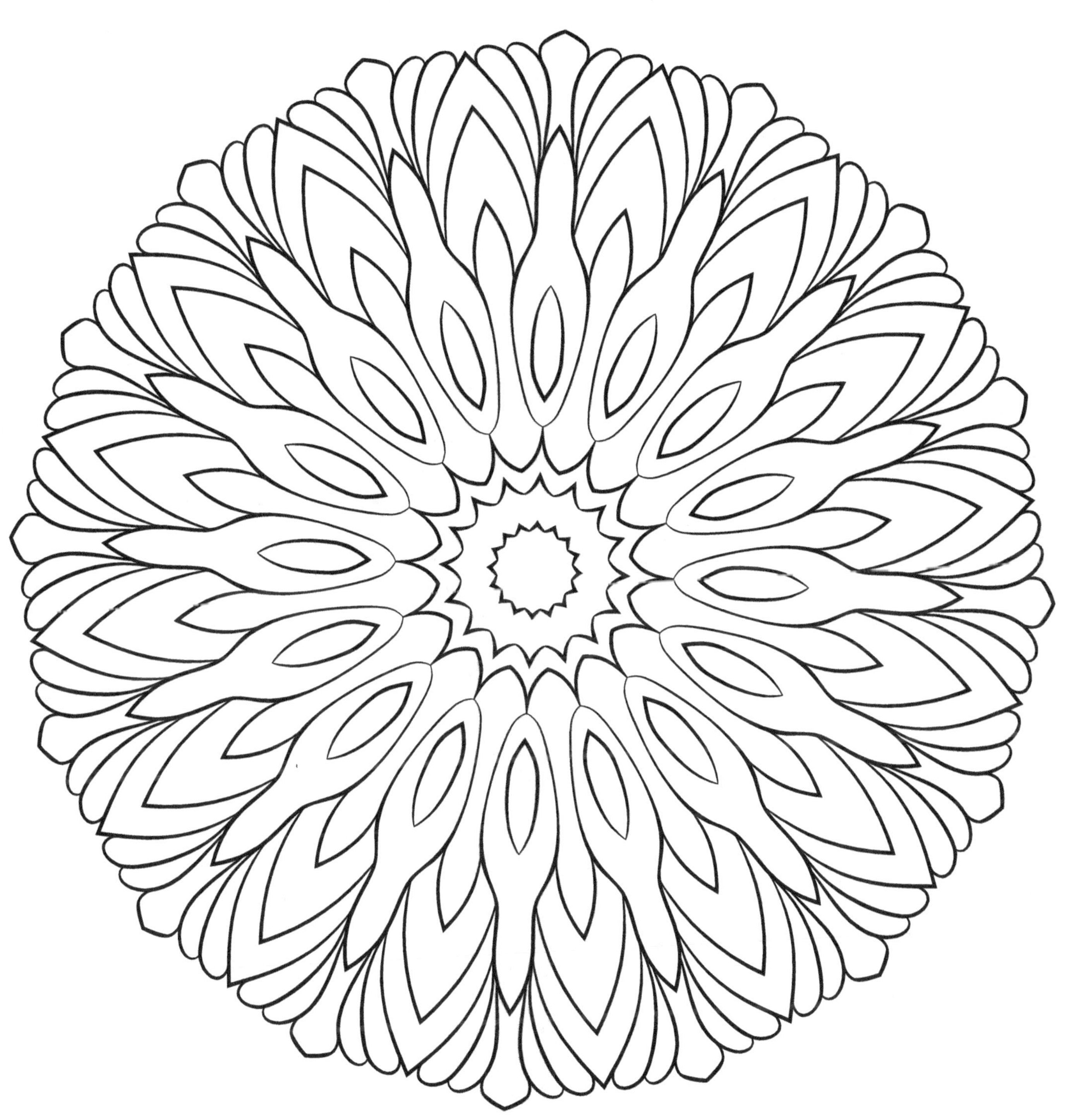

COLORING BOOK

by Little Mary

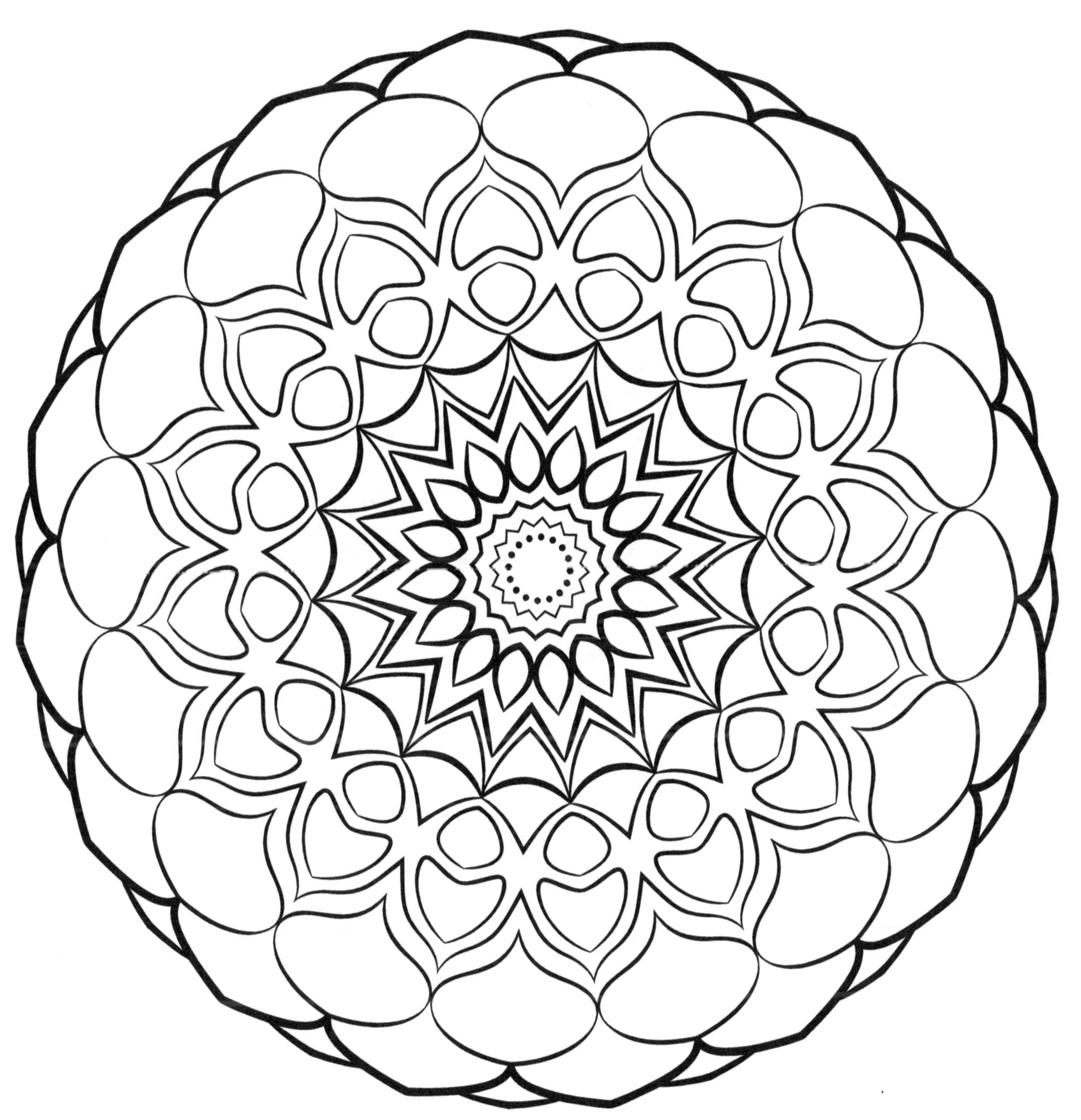

COLORING BOOK

by Little Mary

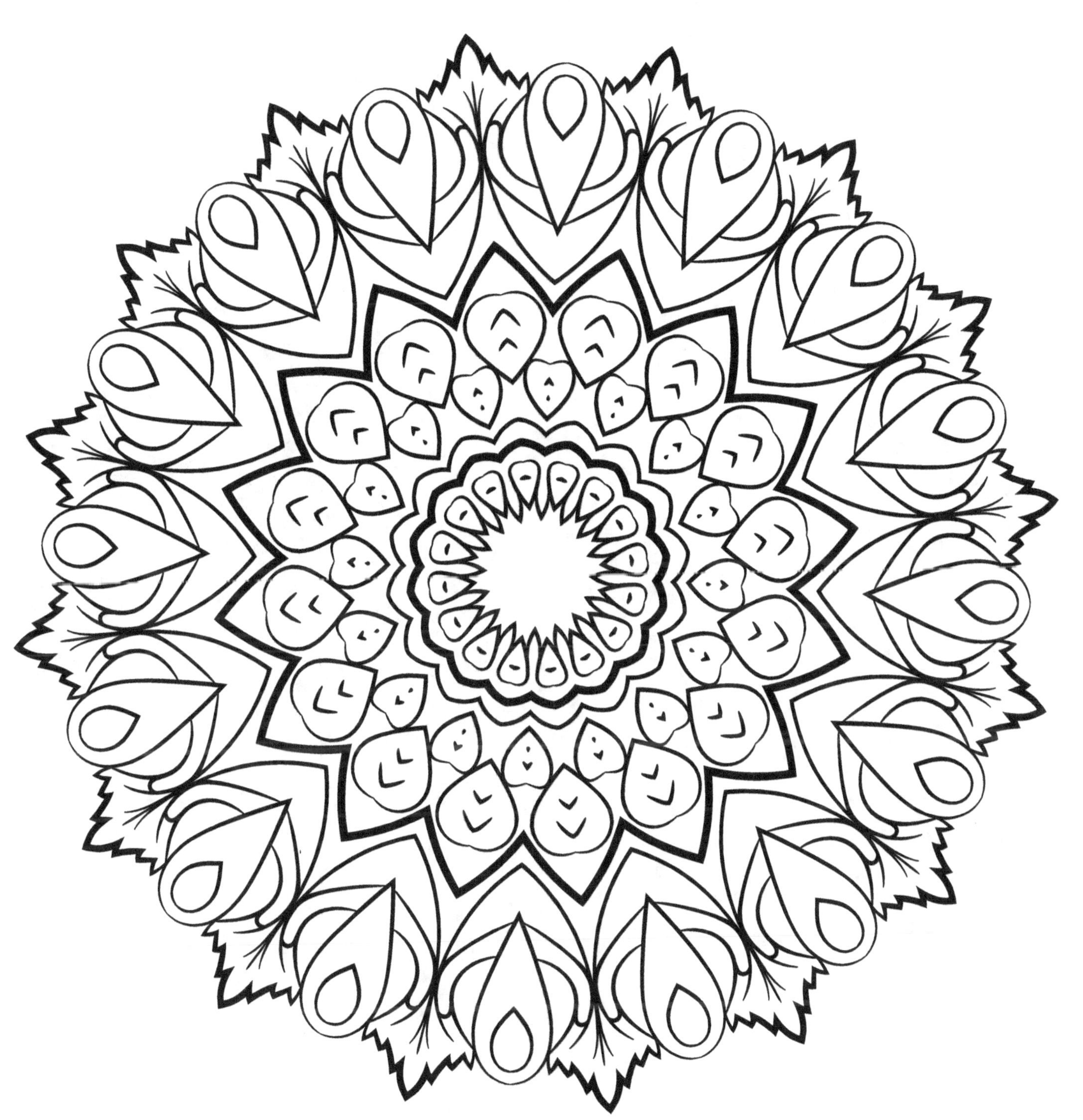

COLORING BOOK

by Little Mary